Self Adjusting Technique

How to gently and affectively self-adjust your neck, back, hips and ribs.

Kalidasa Brown

© 2012 by **Kalidasa Brown**

ISBN
ISBN-13: 978-1469986593

ISBN-10: 1469986590

All Rights Reserved. No part of this publication may be reproduced in any form or by any means, including scanning, photocopying, or otherwise without prior written permission of the copyright holder.

First Printing, 2012

Printed in the United States of America

Liability Disclaimer

This website contains general information about medical conditions and treatments. The information is not advice, and should not be treated as such.

Limitation of warranties

The medical information on this website is provided "as is" without any representations or warranties, express or implied. Kalidasa Brown makes no representations or warranties in relation to the medical information on this website.

Without prejudice to the generality of the foregoing paragraph, Kalidasa Brown does not warrant that:

- the medical information on this website will be constantly available, or available at all; or
- the medical information on this website is complete, true, accurate, up-to-date, or non-misleading.

Terms of Use

You are given a non-transferable, "personal use" license to this book. You cannot distribute it or share it with other individuals.

Also, there are no resale rights or private label rights granted when purchasing this book. In other words, it's for your own personal use only.

Self Adjusting Technique

How to gently and affectively self-adjust your neck, back, hips and ribs.

Table of Contents

Introduction 9
How Self Adjusting Technique was Developed 11
General Cautions 15
Basic Physiology 17
Spinal Misalignments 23
    Physiology of Spinal Misalignments 23
    Finding the Misalignment..24
    The Basic Vertebral Alignment 25
    Persistent Pain in the Neck..29
    Adjusting the Atlas 29
    The Fifth Cervical 35
    Adjusting C5...36
    Adjusting vertebra You Can't Reach 39
    Adjusting the Fifth Lumbar 40
The Ribs 45
    Adjusting the Ribs...46
    The Basic Rib Adjusting Movement 47
    Rib Adjusting Technique 52
    Adjusting the Top Ribs...56
    Adjusting Ribs You Can't Reach 59
    Notes on Adjusting the Ribs 65
    Adjusting the Collar Bone 65
The Lower Back 71
    Stretching the Lower Back...72
    Lower Back Twist Stretch 73
    Deeper Reclining Twist 75
    Lower Back Assisted Ligament Stretch 76
The Sacrum 79
    What a Sacral Misalignment Is 79
    Sacral Adjustment Reclining Twist................................80
    Sacrum Walking Adjustment 84
The Hips and Sacroiliac Joint 91
    Physiology of Hip Misalignments..................................91

- How to Know Which Direction the SI is out 92
- Sacroiliac Adjustment Reclining Twist 93
- SI Reclining Blocking Adjustment 97
- Si Walking Adjustment 100
- Sciatica 109
- The Less Common SI Adjustment 109
- Spinal Compression 111

Muscle Testing 114
- Muscle Testing a Joint 117

The Adrenal Glands 118
- Symptoms of Adrenal Fatigue 125
- 50 Symptoms of Adrenal Fatigue 125
- Adrenal Fatigue Tests 127
- Treatment for the Adrenal Glands 129

Conclusion 134
Contact Me 136
About Kalidasa 138

Introduction

Nine out of ten people will experience back pain some time in their life. Until now the only the only choices back pain sufferers have had was to see a doctor for some drug with serious side effects, see a chiropractor for a scary and possibly painful adjustment, try other techniques like massage that don't really work, or endure the pain while you wait for things to maybe settle down and quit hurting.

Now there is another choice; natural back pain relief with Self Adjusting Technique. Self Adjusting Technique is a way to easily and gently adjust your back, neck, hips and ribs yourself without assistance.

This book describes the method and application of Self Adjusting Technique for these areas. It also contains useful information about how to deal with chronic lower back pain and which often has a biochemical cause.

How Self Adjusting Technique was Developed

Self Adjusting Technique was developed over several years. It started when I had a major illness. Now that I know a lot more about how the various systems of the body work I know why I got so ill. My primary symptom was extreme pain in the gut area. This later developed to include pain in my lower back.

What was happening was the energy systems of my body were depleted to such a degree that major symptoms developed. The back pain was minor compared to the gut pain, so it was not as obvious. I thought that the gut pain and the back pain alternated with much more gut pain. Now I know that I just wasn't aware of the back pain because the gut pain was so much worse!

Eventually I had to have surgery to repair the damage in the gut caused by a blockage in the intestines. The gut pain I had was caused by peristalsis (the constriction and relaxation of the muscles of the intestines that push the contents forward) continuing while the contents were blocked from moving forward. This resulted in damage to the intestines that needed to be repaired surgically.

Medical science knows little about this condition, so they put a label on it to describe a wide variety of symptoms. They call it inflammatory bowel disease. Naturopaths know that there are many causes to this type of condition. One of the causes is depleted energy systems.

These depleted energy systems are also one of the major causes of chronic lower back pain.

A warning here, if the energy systems are depleted, any lower back adjustment, especially a forceful chiropractic adjustment, can result in the back hurting more.

Details on the energy system involved in lower back pain and what you can do to heal this is discussed in the chapter on the adrenal glands. Also, there are two stretches presented that can give some relief.

After the surgery my lower back pain was extreme. My mother was there with me in the recovery room. When I first woke up I had to immediately have her help me bend my knees to relieve the agony my back was in!

The pain persisted, and the only relief I could find when lying on my back was to have my knees supported. Even after going home, I had to get out of bed slowly and walk around for a while until my back 'loosened up.' Finally, I scraped together a little money and went to the chiropractor. I was reluctant because chiropractors always hurt me, but I didn't know what else to do.

I knew a chiropractor, someone I considered a friend, who I thought might help me out. I looked him up and went in for a treatment.

It was my good fortune that he was an activator chiropractor. He used a spring loaded tool called an activator that knocks the various joints back into place. I thought I would be fine after an adjustment, and I could get on with my life, but he told me that I needed to come in at least three times a week for six to eight weeks to get back to 'normal!

I was shocked. I couldn't really afford that one visit because I hadn't been working. I told him of my financial situation hoping he would help me out. But, he couldn't detract from his $175,000 a year practice to give me a few treatments pro bono. It was then that I realized that I would need to get proactive with my health.

I am a yoga teacher, so I knew a little something of physiology and I thought I might be able to figure something out by paying attention to what he did. So, I scraped together another seventy five dollars and went for a second visit. I had to, I was in extreme pain again, pain that persisted even after his adjustment

I paid close attention to where he used the activator tool noting which bones he 'hit' with it. I had this great massage tool, a big 'S' shaped bar with wooden balls at the ends that I was able to use it to pull against the points that he had used the activator on. I reasoned that if I walked around with pressure against the places where he used his activator that the joints might move back to where they belonged. And, it worked!

Every morning I would drag myself painfully out of bed, get my massage tool and walk around the house for forty-five minutes or more pulling everything back into place.

Eventually I worked out other easier ways to do the adjustments. Then I found several ways to do some of the same adjustments. The ribs were the hardest to figure out, but I found a way and refined it to the current easy methods.

Next, I started trying it on friends of mine. That went so well that I was able to develop an adjusting practice for people who were afraid of the forcing, cracking and pain that chiropractors may cause. Later, I started teaching my clients how to do the adjustments themselves, and Self Adjusting Technique was born.

General Cautions

While Self Adjusting Technique is very gentle, and it is almost impossible to hurt yourself, it is good to be cautious. Consulting your doctor is a good idea. Consider this the obligatory disclaimer to utilize Self Adjusting Technique at your own risk.

If you have a serious injury, if there is damage to the area you are adjusting, if the ligaments are extremely weak, if the area is hyper mobile (the joint moves very easily or all the time), extra caution may be warranted. These are conditions I come across and treat successfully in my practice with supplements.

The only situation I have ever found where no adjustment of any kind should be done is with a herniated disc. When certain energy systems are depleted, adjustments to the lower back may result in more discomfort. This issue can be easily cleared up with dietary corrections and supplements which are discussed in the section on the adrenal glands.

The main thing to watch for when doing any of the self adjusting techniques is pain. Pain should always be listened to no matter what you are doing! Pain is your body telling you that something is wrong, and whatever you are doing that is causing the pain should be stopped immediately.

This doesn't always apply as in 'good' pain like when you stretch out. The pain to watch for is the pain that causes you to resist. It is the tensing from this resistance that can and often does cause injury.

If there is already an injury, pain will be a major warning! Re-injuries can take up to ten times longer to heal than the original injury even when using holistic treatment. I don't know how many injuries I have treated that happened as a result of ignoring pain.

The adjusting techniques presented in this book don't involve stretching rather they are gentle manipulations with movement.

Basic Physiology

Following is a brief explanation of the physiology of the areas that are covered in this book, the spine, hips and ribs. Parts of this information are repeated in the appropriate sections for convenience.

The spine is divided into five sections. The neck area is called the cervical spine with seven vertebras. The part of the spine associated with the chest cavity is called the thoracic spine which has twelve vertebras. The lower back or the lumbar spine has five vertebras.

The sacrum is a triangular shaped group of five fused vertebra. At the bottom of the spine is the coccyx or tail bone which is formed of fused vestigial vertebra. The usual number of coccygeal vertebra is four, but it can vary from one to as many as seven.

Vertebras are the individual bones that form the backbone. They each have several projections for connecting to other bones and for muscle attachments. They each have a hole through them for the spinal cord to pass through. The obvious part of the vertebra which protrudes at the very back of the spine is called the Spinous process. This is a longer projection that has many muscles attached to it.

The hips are a bowl shaped bone. It forms a joint with the spine in the back called the sacroiliac joint or the SI. This joint is formed along the side of the sacrum where it articulates or forms a joint with a ridge of bone of the hip called the posterior iliac spine, the hip point in back. A misalignment of the SI joint is a major cause of chronic lower back pain.

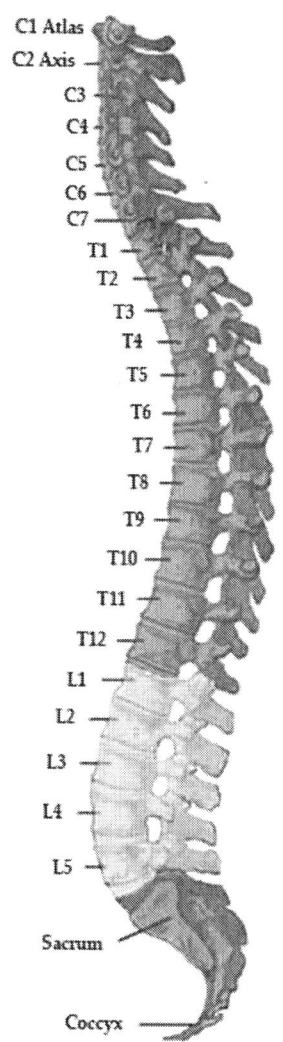

Sections of the Spine

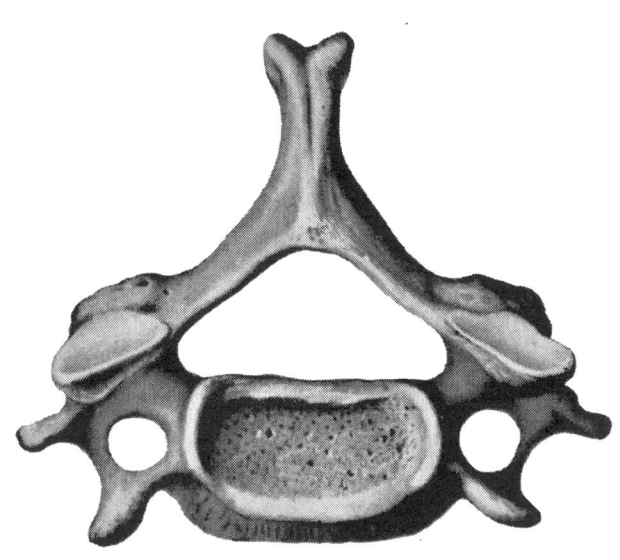

A Typical Vertebral Structure with its Prominent Spinous Process which is Pointing Up in this Photo

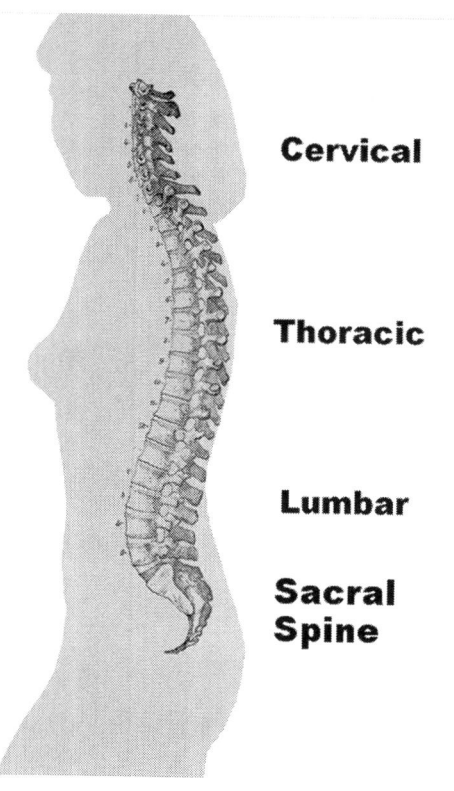

The Location of the Various Parts of the Spine in the Body

The prominent hip bones in the front are called the anterior (front of the body) superior (upper) iliacus spine (describes the ridge of bone) or ASIS. The hip bones in the back are called the posterior (back of the body) superior iliacus spine or PSIS. The ischium or sit bones are at the bottom just back of the center of the hip structure.

The sacrum sits down into the hip structure in the back. This is where the weight of the upper body is transferred to the lower body, first into the hip structure, and from there into the legs.

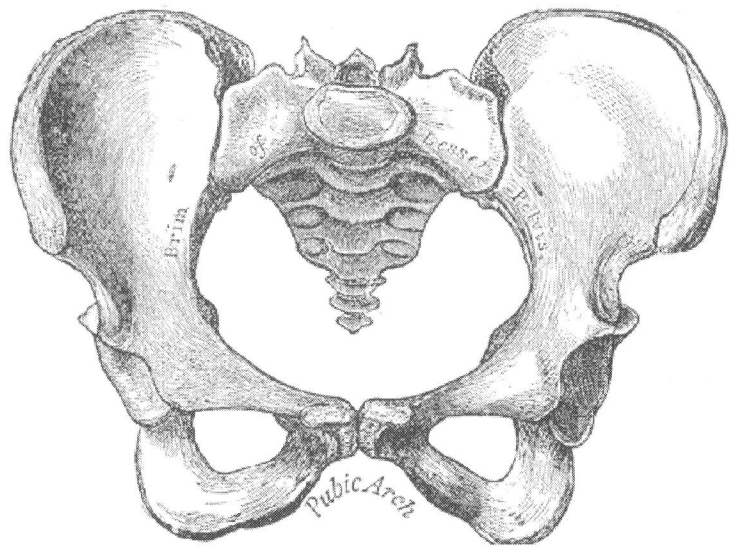

Hips and Sacrum Front View

There are twelve ribs which articulate with or form a joint with the twelve thoracic vertebras. The uppermost ribs connect with the sternum in the front. Lower down they connect with each other to the side of the diaphragm. The lower two ribs don't connect in the front and are called floating ribs.

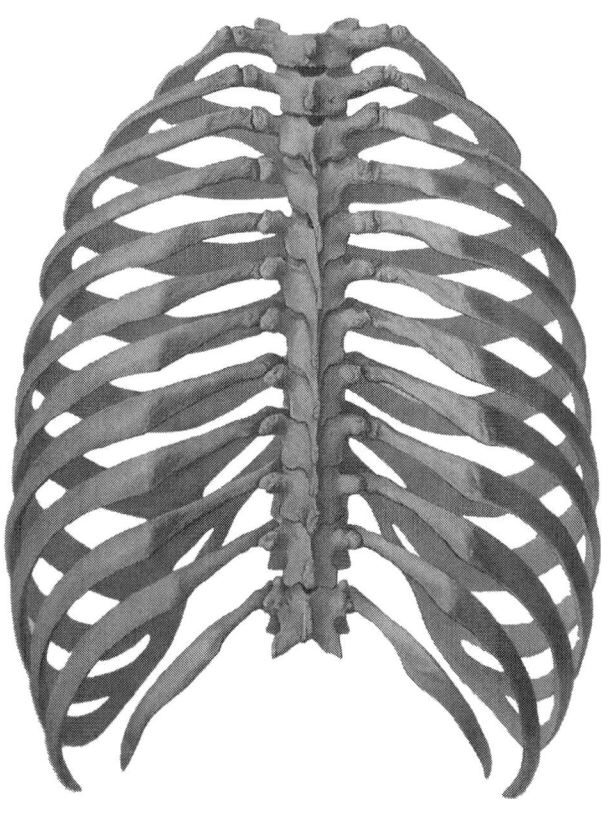

Ribs and Thoracic Spine Back View

Spinal Misalignments

The individual vertebra each have a bony part which protrudes at the back called the Spinous process. This is the obvious part of the spine, the bones that show in the back. The Spinous process will be involved in all vertebral adjustments.

Physiology of Spinal Misalignments

The most common misalignment in the spine happens when one or more vertebras rotate to one side or the other. Think of the Spinous process as pointing more to one side or the other rather than straight back. This is a rotational misalignment of a spinal vertebra. These rotational misalignments are common with one or more being somewhere in the spine

There is almost always a rotational misalignment somewhere in the spine which usually goes unnoticed. You can probably find examples of these misalignments in your neck or back by feeling for them. Just press around in your neck or back and you will most likely find some tight or tender muscles on one side or the other of the vertebra.

Usually one side will be tenderer than the other. These minor misalignments aren't usually noticed because they *are* minor and they adjust themselves as you twist and move about in your normal movements throughout the day. In a way, Self Adjusting Technique is an extension of the natural way the body is doing these realignments all the time.

Misalignments can happen for many reasons. You could

sleep in a strange position and wake with a stiff neck. You could fall or bang yourself in such a way that you knock something out of alignment. Sometimes muscles tense up, usually from stress, causing a misalignment. These stress induced misalignments are the ones that are more likely to bother you.

A simple misalignment is when one or more vertebra rotates to the same side. Sometimes though one vertebra will rotate to one side while one above or below rotates the other way. A fixation is when this happens and they lock in place. You can even have several vertebras in a row each rotating to alternate sides. This can be the most uncomfortable misalignment; sometimes it can be quite painful.

Finding the Misalignment

It is important to find where the misalignment is as well as which side the vertebra has rotated to so that you can know which way to do the adjustment. This technique is so gentle though that it is very difficult to hurt yourself, even if you do the adjustment the wrong way.

You first need to find where the spine is misaligned. Often this is obvious because of the pain or discomfort. The method of finding the various misalignments presented in this book is to feel for the discomfort.

When looking for a misalignment in the spine, note which side is most sore. This is probably the side the vertebra has rotated to. This is an important step, so take your time and feel around. Get to know what is really going on.

If the soreness is on the right side of the vertebra, then the rotation is most likely to the right, which means that it needs to rotate back to the left.

Note that just because a vertebra is physically more to one side or the other relative to the rest of the spine doesn't necessarily mean that it has rotated to that side. Everyone has at least a little scoliosis in the spine, that is, a curve to one side or the other. I have seen spines that curve so sharply that all of a sudden a vertebra is a half inch or more to one side of the rest of the spine.

Realignment with this technique can be a great relief for people with moderate to major scoliosis as vertebra often rotates out of alignment because of the curvature in the spine.

The muscles will tend to tense up on the side of the vertebral rotation which causes the soreness. Pressing on the muscles tends to release them like a massage might. These muscles don't necessarily need a massage to release enough for the realignment, but massage can help when there is a lot of stiffness and the adjustment technique doesn't seem to work. You could get a massage, or even work the muscles yourself.

The Basic Vertebral Alignment

The basic technique for adjusting any vertebra involves a little pressure into the bunched up muscles just to the side of the Spinous process, the side that is tender, the side the vertebra rotated to, along with a twist in the opposite direction of the vertebral rotation.

As you twist, all the vertebras rotate the same way you are twisting. The pressure to the side of the Spinous process releases the muscle and assists that vertebra to rotate back into position as you turn. In most cases only four ounces or less of pressure is needed to bring vertebra back into alignment.

More pressure may be needed in some cases. Start with a light pressure though as you are less likely to cause more discomfort if you are working the vertebra the wrong way.

Let's look at the third cervical as an example. It is about two and a half to three inches below the base of the skull.

Suppose it is very tender on the left side, but not so tender on the right. To adjust, take your right hand behind the back of your neck and gently pull on the left side of the Spinous process. Use whichever finger that is easiest for you to pull into the muscles just to the left of the Spinous process.

Gently pressing into the muscle releases the muscles on the left side and encourages the Spinous process to the right.

From a forward facing position drop your chin so the vertebra is a little more pronounced. While continuing to press into the muscles which are to the left side of the Spinous process, slowly turn your head to the left. Continue to press into the area just to the side of the Spinous process allowing your finger to follow along. Remember, it only takes about four ounces of pressure to affect the adjustment. Release and turn your head back to center.

This is the basic technique for all the vertebras. A little pressure to encourage the vertebra in the direction it needs to move, and a rotation of the spine opposite to the side you are pulling or pushing on. You could just as easily use the right hand and push on the vertebra if that works better for you.

There are some variations for adjusting the first cervical at the top of the neck, the fifth cervical which is deeper in and harder to adjust as well as the adjustment for the fifth lumbar in the lower back. These are covered later.

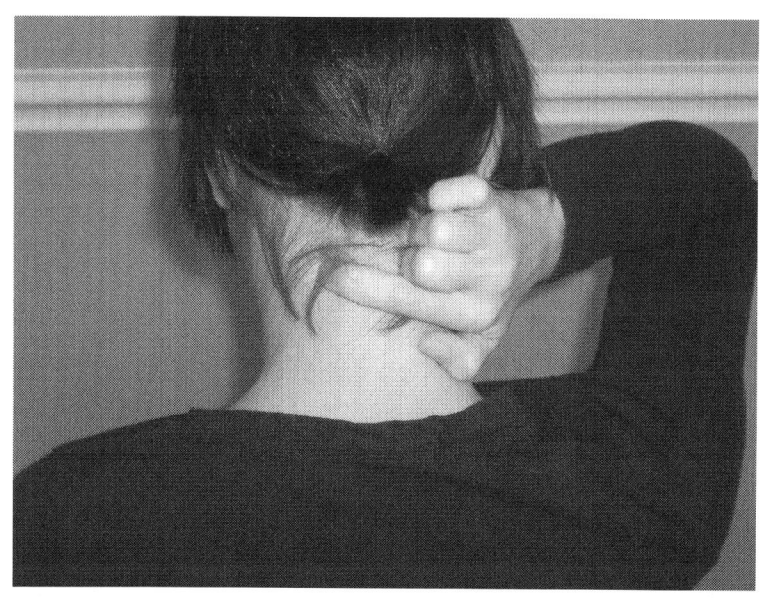

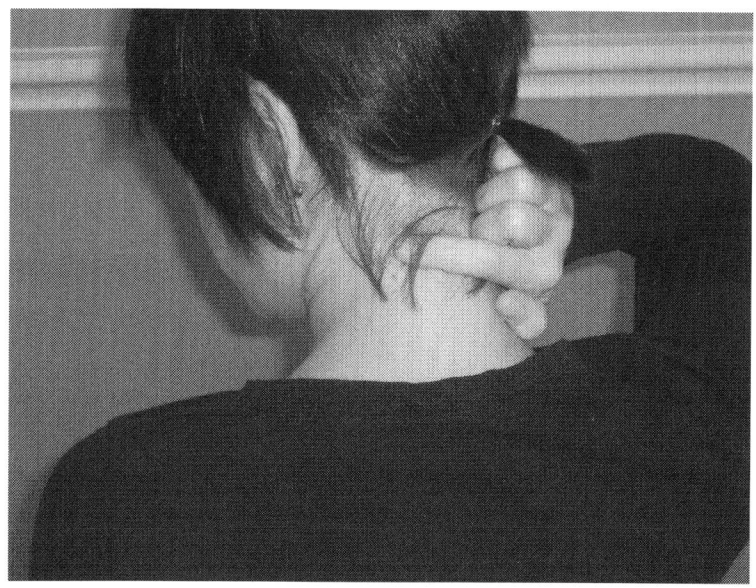

Adjusting Example: C3

Persistent Pain in the Neck

A very common problem in the neck is tension that runs up into the neck from the ribs in the upper back. These misaligned ribs can cause tension all the way up into the neck, and when combined with a misalignment in the neck can cause a lot of pain in the neck area. It may not feel like the ribs in the upper back are involved, but they often are.

Tension headaches in the back of the head can be caused by this combination as well. If you do the neck adjustment and the neck area still hurts, adjust the upper three or four ribs on that side as well. See the section on adjusting the ribs.

Adjusting the Atlas

The atlas is at the very top of the neck. It is the connection between the spine and the skull. Most of the rotation for the head happens with C1 rotating around on C2. Because of this it is often out of alignment.

It is a very wide vertebra which needs two adjustments on each side even if it doesn't seem like it is out of alignment on both sides. Besides, the technique is so gentle it is more of a massage than an adjustment, so an extra adjustment is more like a little massage.

The first part of the adjustment is to press into the muscle group that is further out from the vertebra than you would press when doing the basic method. The point is about an inch and a half from the Spinous process. There is a little depression there to the side of the muscles that run alongside the vertebra. Push or pull the area to the left as you turn your head to the left. Next, move your finger into the muscles that attach to the Spinous process as in the basic technique and do the adjustment there. That is, pull or press the Spinous process to the left and turn your head to the right. Repeat the two steps on the left side.

The adjustment can be done by pulling the vertebra or by pushing it as you do the movement. Both are shown in the following photos.

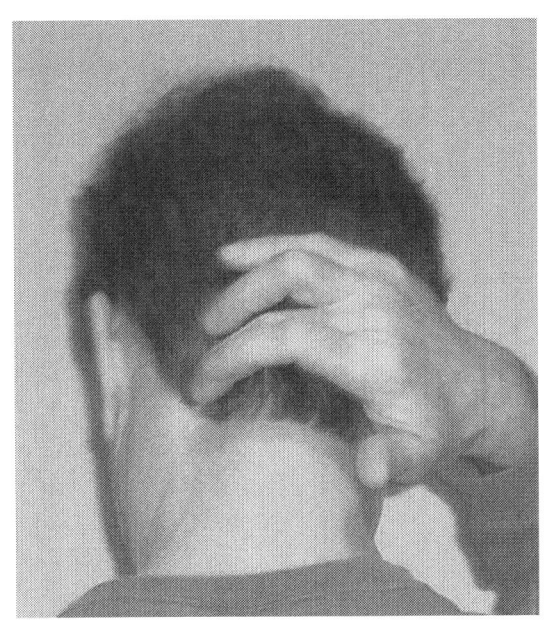

The First C1 is Further Out, Just below the Base of the Skull

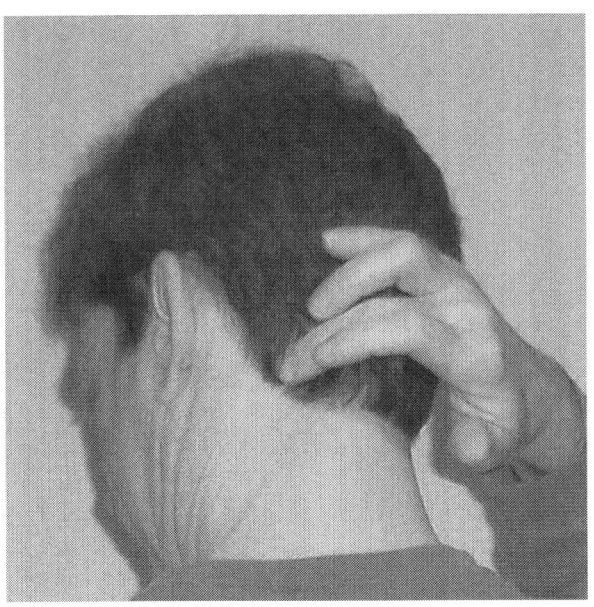

Drop Your Chin and Turn the Head

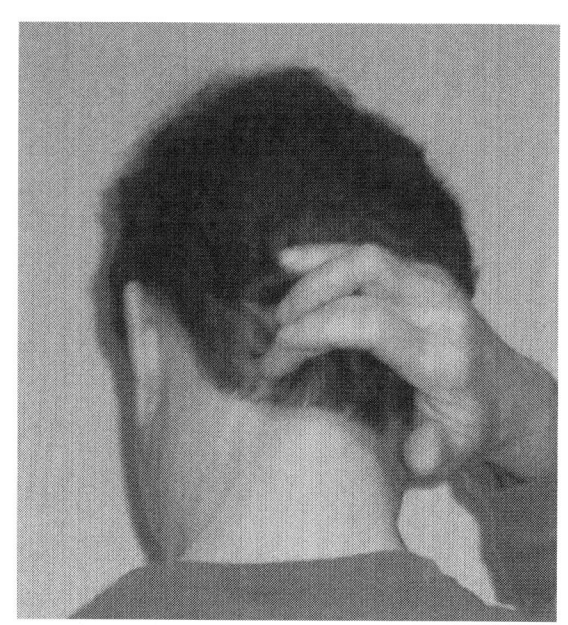

Move Your Finger in Closer

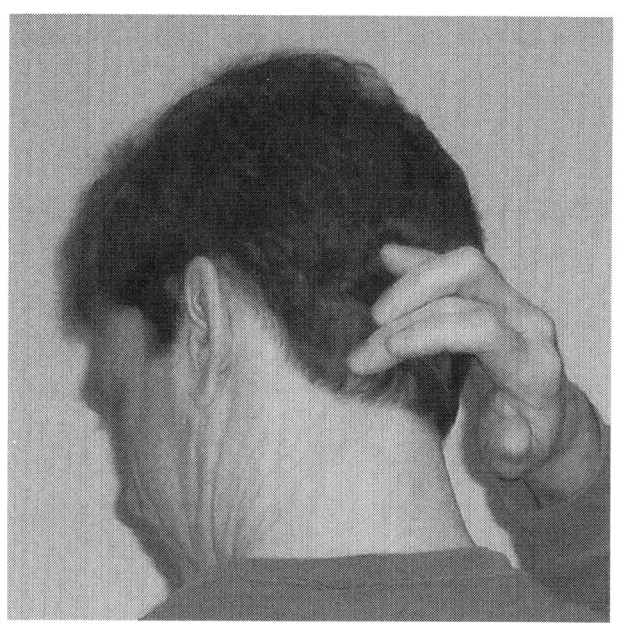

And Adjust Again

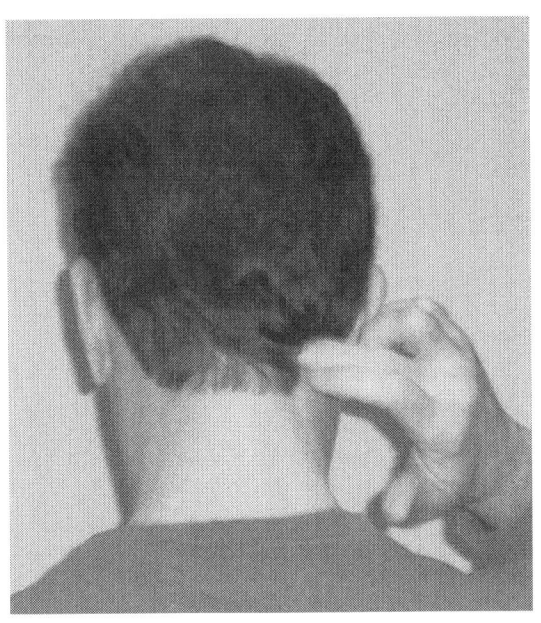

Push Method is the Same, Push Further out First

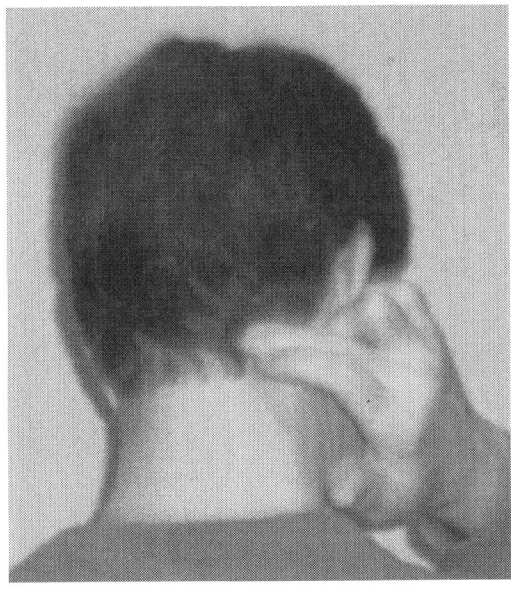

Keep Your Chin Down and Turn the Head

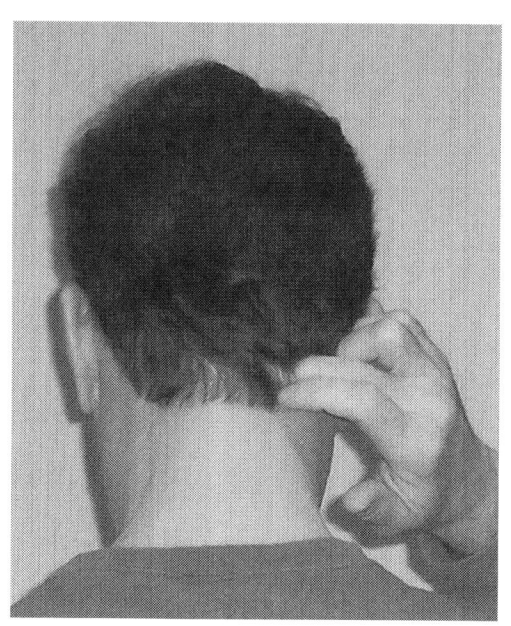

Move the Finger in Slightly

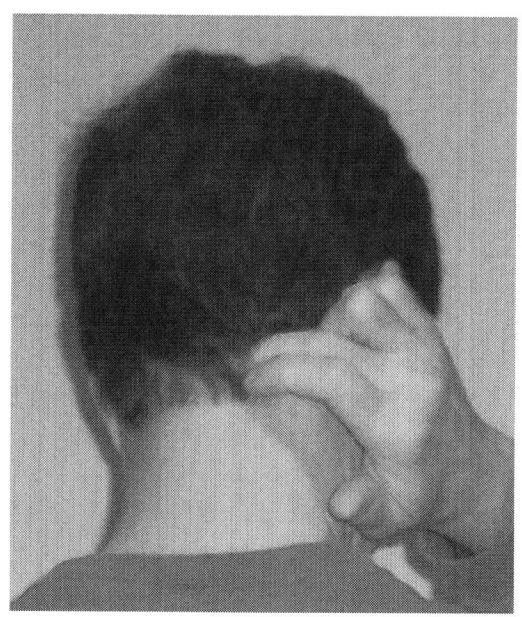

Apply Some Pressure and Turn the Head

The Fifth Cervical

The fifth cervical is chronically out of alignment in most people. The reason for this has to do with the Vagus nerve which is a thick nerve bundle that runs down from the brain stem on either side of the spine to C5. Smaller nerve bundles then branch off into different areas of the body. Many of these nerve fibers go into the gut area where they regulate the body's sugar handling mechanism.

Digestion breaks down all carbohydrates into sugars. This includes the slower digesting carbohydrates like fruits, vegetables and whole grains. This slow method of releasing sugar is the process that the body is designed for.

Faster digesting carbohydrates like ground up grains, steel cut or quick oats, white rice, sugar, honey, maple syrup, dried fruits, fruit juice and sometimes sweet fruits like bananas, oranges and red apples are the carbohydrates that cause problems. These all release sugar into the blood stream quickly which causes the metabolism to react rigorously to keep blood sugar levels within a certain range.

The information needed to keep blood sugar balanced is processed through Vagus nerve. A back up happens with all this extra information going into Vagus nerve from the smaller branches at C5. It's like several freeways merging together during rush hour.

The backup causes tension in the muscles which pulls C5 out of alignment. With continued consumption of processed foods and sugar, C5 will chronically be out of alignment.

Eventually the disc between C5 and C6 will bulge. This bulging disc presses into a large group of nerves that runs from the neck down the arm and into the hand. A tingling sometimes happens in the arm and hand that can become painful.

Sometimes this is mistaken for carpal tunnel syndrome. If you have this sensation in the arm and hand, or if C5 just doesn't want to go back into place, you will need to stop eating the fast metabolizing carbohydrates for several weeks before you can affectively adjust C5.

To demonstrate this for clients with this problem, I will adjust C5 and hold it in place with my finger. It only takes a few seconds before the tingling in their arm and hand subsides almost completely. The sensation returns almost immediately after I let go.

Adjusting C5

C5 is the deepest vertebra in the neck, and is hard to get to for an adjustment. Sometimes it can even be difficult to find. To expose it you need to drop your chin down as far as you can. Keep your chin down while rotating your head for the adjustment.

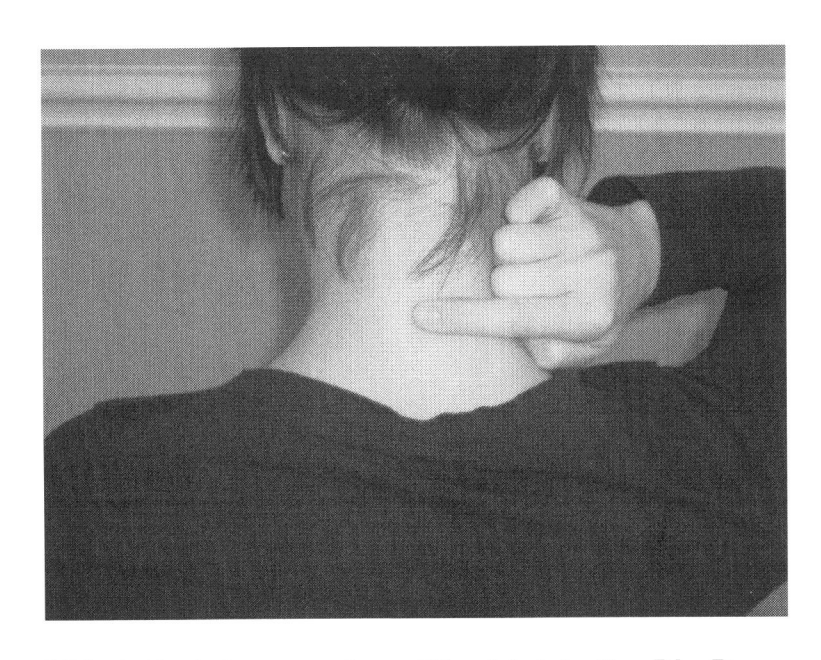

**C5 is 3 Vertebras up from T1 which is the Big Bump
It is Hard to Find Unless You Drop Your Chin as Far
as You Can**

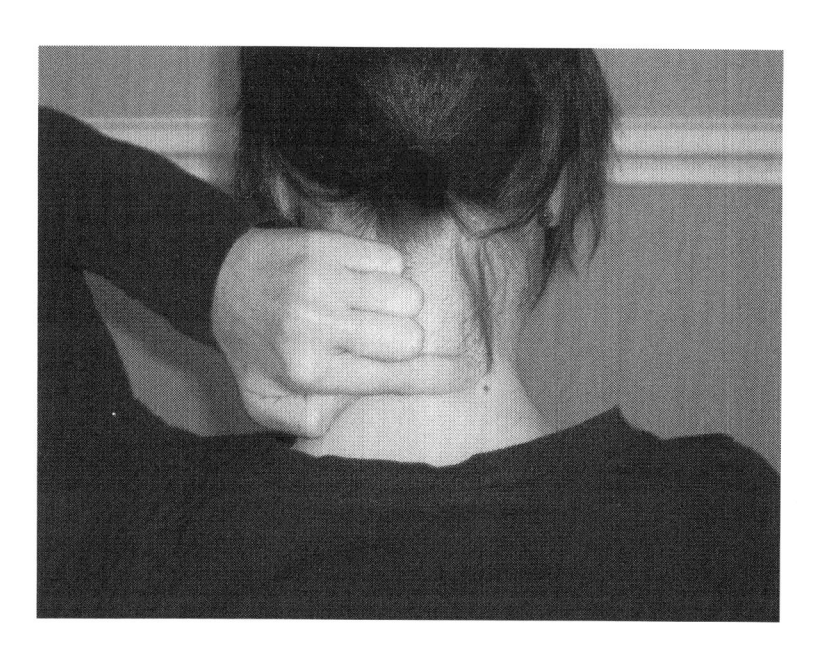

Take the Chin All the Way down Press on the Side of C5

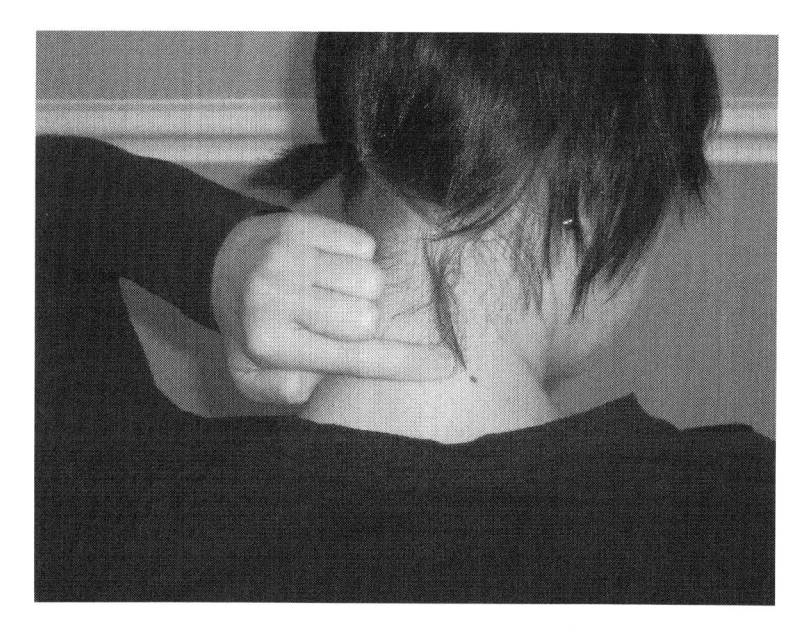

Keep Your Chin Down as You Turn the Head

Adjusting vertebra You Can't Reach

There are two ways to adjust areas you can't reach. One is to have someone help you. Have them press around in the area that is tender as you guide them to find the spot that needs adjusting. Then have them push against the side of vertebra as you rotate your head or torso. They may need to get used to following the vertebra as you turn.

The other way to adjust vertebra you can't reach can be done with a massage tool. The tool that works perfectly for this is the S Hook Self Massager. They can be found in many health food stores or online.

Hook the tool around your waist and use the little ball at the end of the tool to press into the correct area to find where the adjustment is needed. Then, you can use the tool to push against the side of the vertebra as you rotate it back into alignment.

The massage tool pictured here is one of the least expensive. It's a great tool to have around for self massage too.

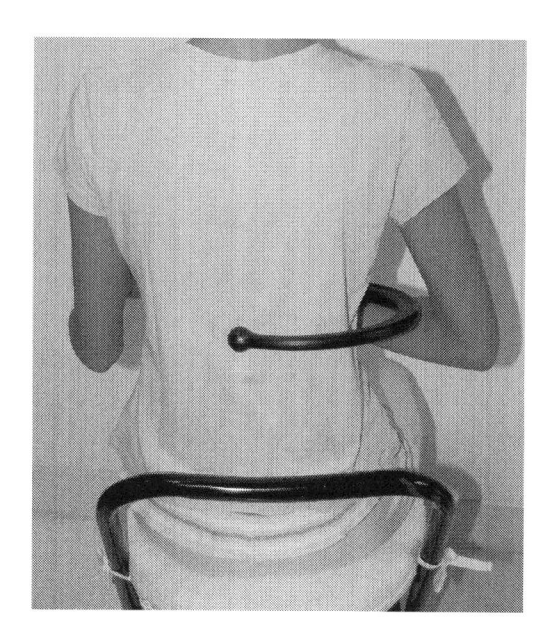

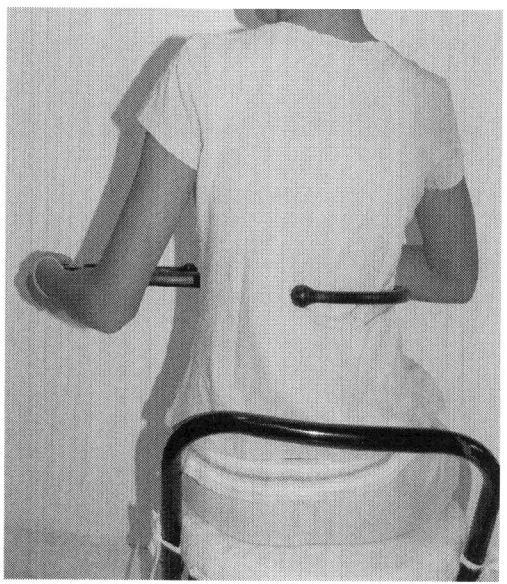

Adjusting the Back with a Massage Tool

Adjusting the Fifth Lumbar

You can find the fifth lumbar by finding L4 first. The hip bones in the back which are about one and a half to two inches out from the spine are in a line with L4. L5 is the next one down with the sacrum below that.

L5 is often involved with lower back pain. The lumbar spine consists of five vertebras. They rotate as you twist like the rest of the vertebra, but L5 rotates in the opposite direction of your twist. This may not seem right, but the fact is that when you twist to the right, the fifth lumbar vertebra rotates to the left. Consequently, the fifth lumbar is the only one that needs a special technique.

For the most part, when adjusting the back you only need a small twist, it really doesn't take much at all. L5 needs a deep twist though. Do this adjustment in the same basic way, but twist as far as you can by pulling deeply into the twist. The best way to do this is to sit in a chair with a high back perhaps with arms that you can hold onto to pull yourself deeply into the twist. Or, sit on the chair sideways and use the back of the chair to pull yourself into the twist. You can do this adjustment by pushing on L5 with a finger or with the massage tool.

To locate L5, first find the two hip points in the back, where the right finger is pointing. These hip bones are on the same level as L4, so the next one down is L5, where the left finger is pointing in the next photo.

The adjustment for L5 usually takes a deep twist unless your spine is very flexible.

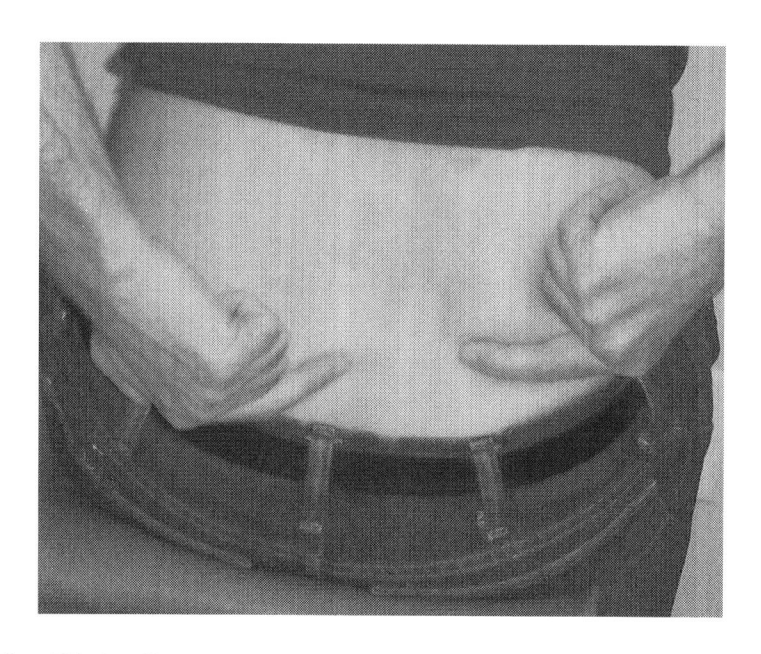

**The Right finger Points to PSIS, the Hip Bone in Back
The Left Finger Points to L5**

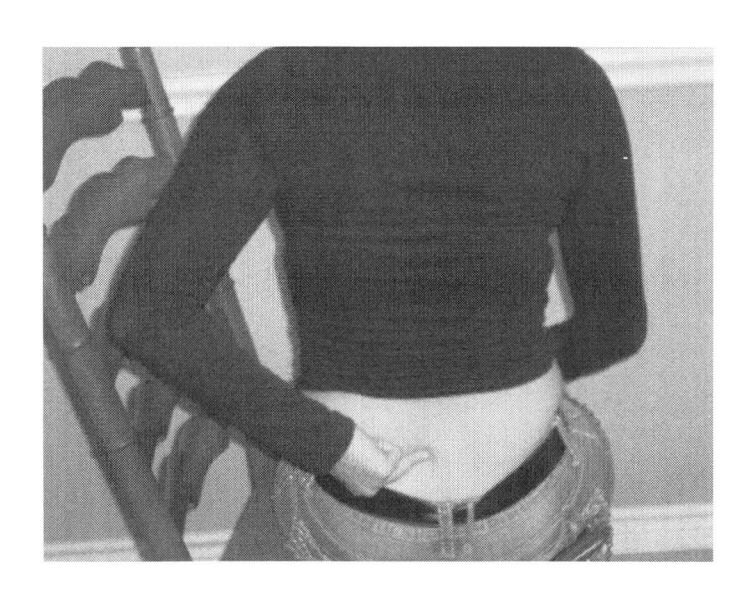

L5 Adjustment -- Pressure on the Side of the Vertebra

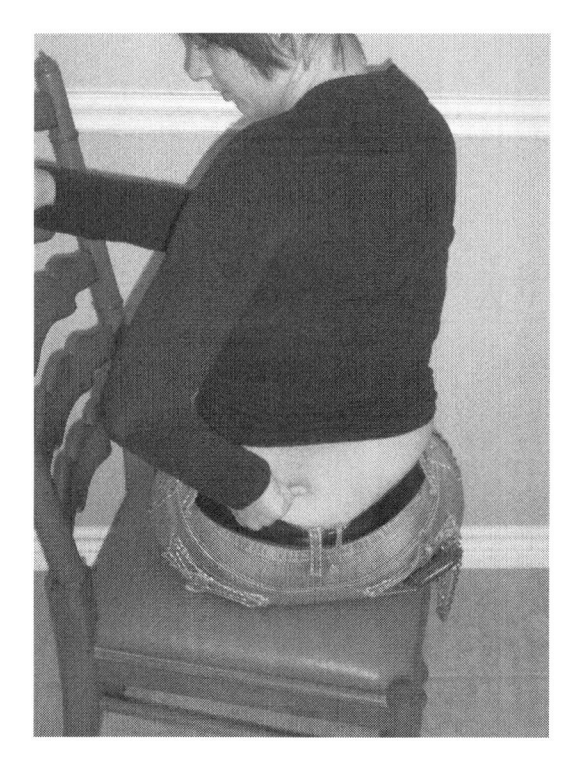

L5 Adjustment, deep twist pulling on chair back

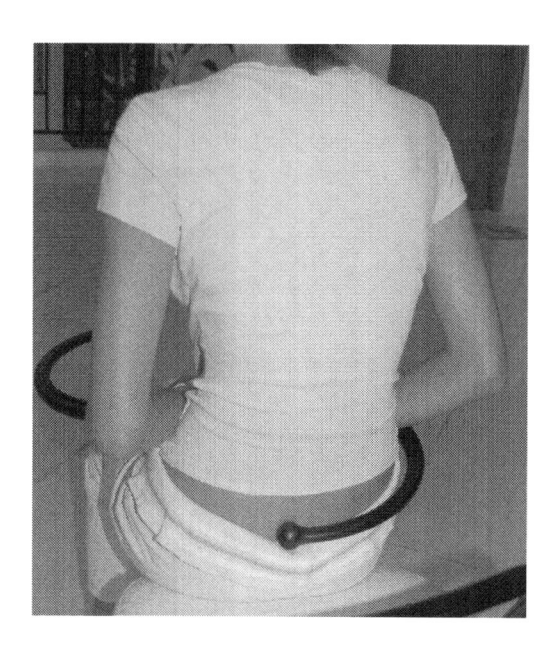

Using a Massage Tool for L5 Adjustment

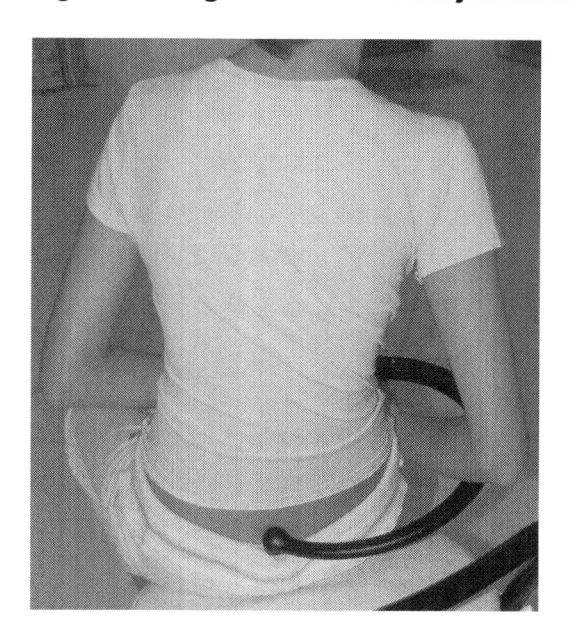

Use a Chair Back to Pull into the Twist While Applying Pressure with the Massage Tool

The Ribs

There are twelve ribs on either side of the spine that articulate with or form a joint with the twelve thoracic vertebras. (Thoracic refers to the chest cavity.) The top ten ribs come together in the chest area attaching to the sternum in the upper chest. They also come together below the sternum to the side of the diaphragm area. All of these connections form joints and can become misaligned.

People often think of the area at the top of the back or around the shoulder blade as having 'knots' in the muscles. It may be true that the muscles 'knot up,' but many of these bunched up muscles are caused by one or more ribs being out of alignment.

Or, the bunched up muscles can pull the ribs out of alignment. It often surprises people to find that there is a rib at the very top of the shoulder, the first rib. This rib is often out of alignment, and people often write it off as one of these knots thinking that this is just normal tightness.

It is true that this is an area where tension from the stress of life can cause problems. Misaligned ribs can be a big part of the tension, tightness and pain in the back.

Sometimes a rib will go out of alignment in such a way that it is hard to breath. A deep breath can even be painful with some rib misalignments. Putting these ribs back into alignment can be a great relief. You can easily tell if you were successful in putting the rib back in alignment because you will be able to take a deep breath again.

Often there are several ribs out in the area of pain. Keep adjusting the ribs above and below the area until you are comfortable again.

The ribs tend to go out in a specific direction. The upper eight ribs almost always move up when they go out of alignment, so they need to adjust in a downward direction. The lower four ribs almost always move down and need to move up for realignment.

This isn't always the case, but you will be pretty safe to assume that is what is needed. If you don't get relief, try adjusting in the other direction.

Adjusting the Ribs

Like many of the self adjusting methods, adjusting the ribs requires movement. The basic movement is the same for all the ribs though the first two don't usually need the whole movement.

It is much easier to learn how to do the movement before doing the adjustment because it is an unusual movement that often requires practice. Doing a strange movement and applying the right pressure on the rib at the same time can be very difficult. Most of the ribs will go in if the movement is not done precisely, but there are some that simply won't go in unless you do the movement exactly.

The Basic Rib Adjusting Movement

The direction of the movement depends on which side the rib is on that you are adjusting. In this case, we'll say that you are adjusting a rib on the right side.

The movement starts with a flexion of the torso, or rolling your body forward. Then, while your body is still rolled forward, rotate your upper body to the left side. Stay rolled forward while rotating back to the right. Stay twisted to the right as you bring your torso back upright and arch your back as much as you comfortably can. Stay arched as you turn back forward and release.

To break it down into steps, for adjusting a rib on the right side:
1. Roll your upper body forward.
2. Maintain the forward roll and twist the torso to the left.
3. Maintain the forward roll while you twist to the right.
4. Maintain the twist to the right side and bring the torso upright and arch the back.
5. Maintain the arch and turn back forward.

If you are adjusting a rib on the left side of the body, just change the lefts and rights. Breaking this down into steps:
1. Roll your torso forward, flexion.
2. Maintain the forward roll and twist the torso to the right.
3. Maintain the forward roll while you twist to the left.
4. Maintain the twist to the left side and bring the torso upright and arch the back.
5. Maintain the arch and turn back forward.

Practice this several times. Some of the movements may be completely alien to you. Also, it can be hard to concentrate on how to move your body while pressing the rib.

People tend to do all kinds of variations because they just aren't used to staying rolled forward while twisting. The tendency is to bring the torso back up while rotating.

After you have gotten the movement down you can push the rib in the appropriate direction while doing the movements.

You can find the ribs that need an adjustment by pressing around in the area that is uncomfortable. The ribs are higher, pronounced and hard; the bones are separated by a lower space in between the more pronounced ribs, kind of like hills and valleys.

The place to push is between the ribs and either down or up on the bone depending on which way it is out.

For example, if you are adjusting the fourth rib, you will find the rib bone, and then notice the tender area above the rib. You may experience it as a knot in the muscle. Press down on this rib near the spine to adjust.

A second adjustment may be needed a little further out from the spine.

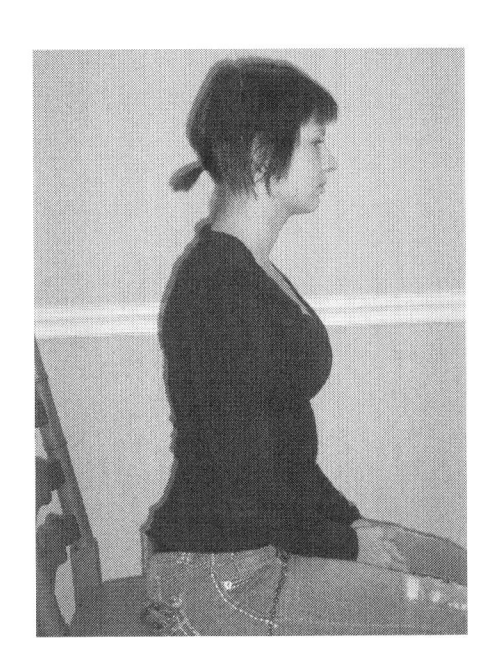

Rib Movement Starting Position

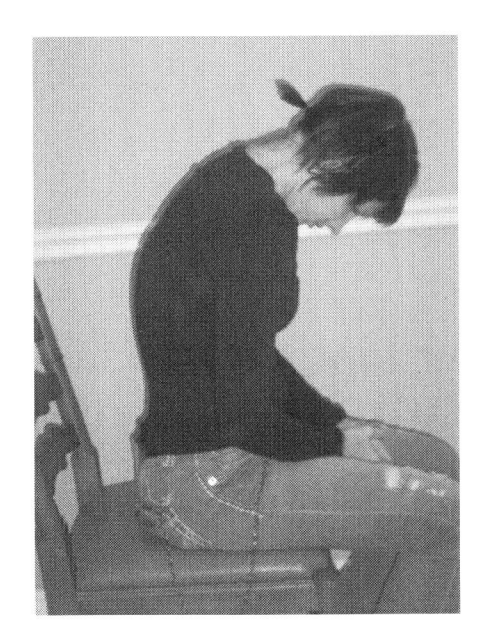

Roll Forward

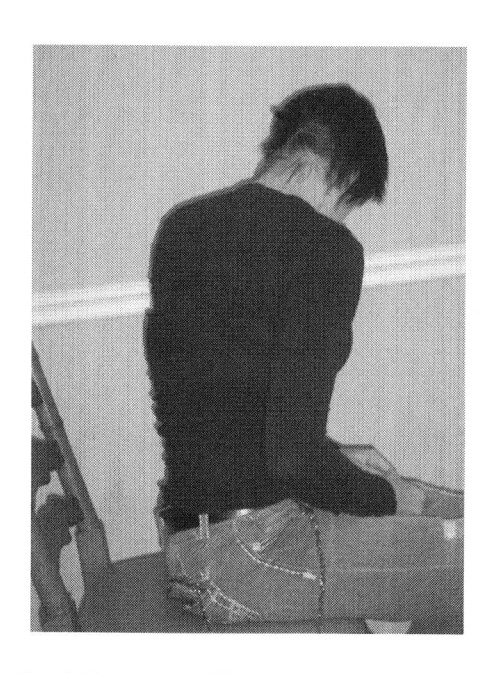

Stay Rolled Forward While Rotating to the Left

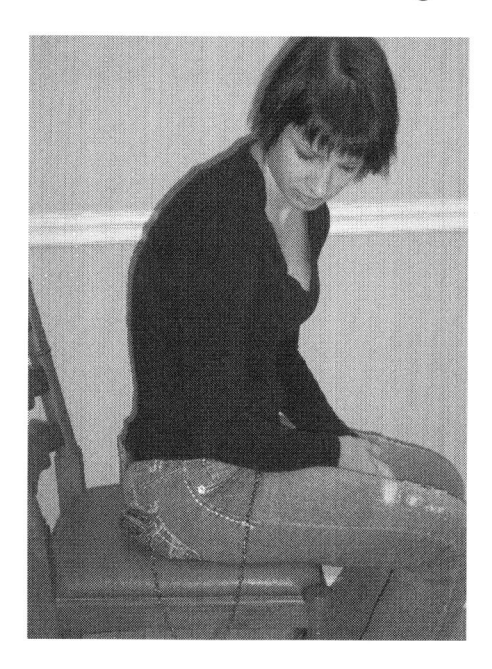

Stay Rolled Forward While Rotating to the Right

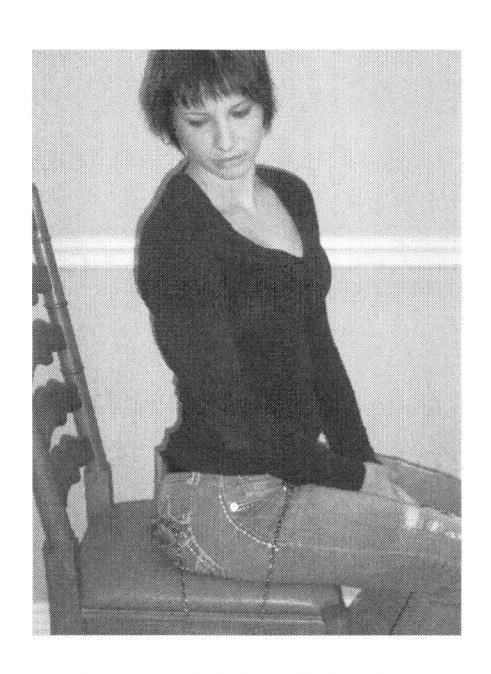

Stay Rotated to the Right While Coming Up and Arching the Back

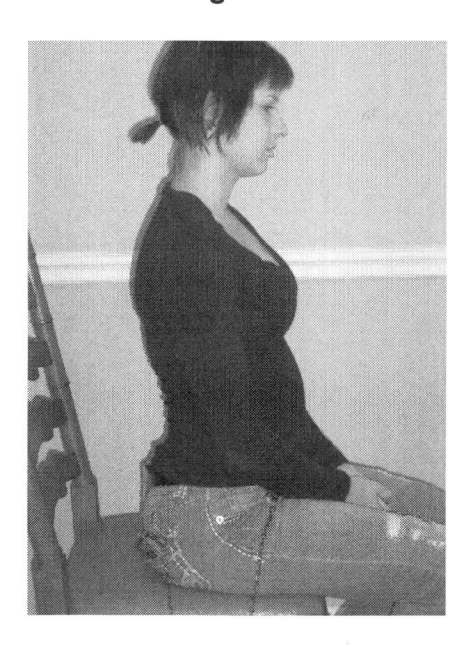

Keep the Arch While Turning Back Forward

Rib Adjusting Technique

As mentioned before, the direction you push the rib will be mostly dependent on which rib you are adjusting. The upper eight ribs tend to go out in an upward direction, so they will need to move down. The last four ribs tend to go out in a downward direction, so they will need to move up.

This can vary, but the adjustment is not going to damage anything if you are pressing the rib in the wrong direction, even if you try to adjust it several times. Consider that the rib may need to move in the other direction if it seems like it isn't going in. This is rare though.

Adjusting a rib in front uses the same movements as the ribs in back.

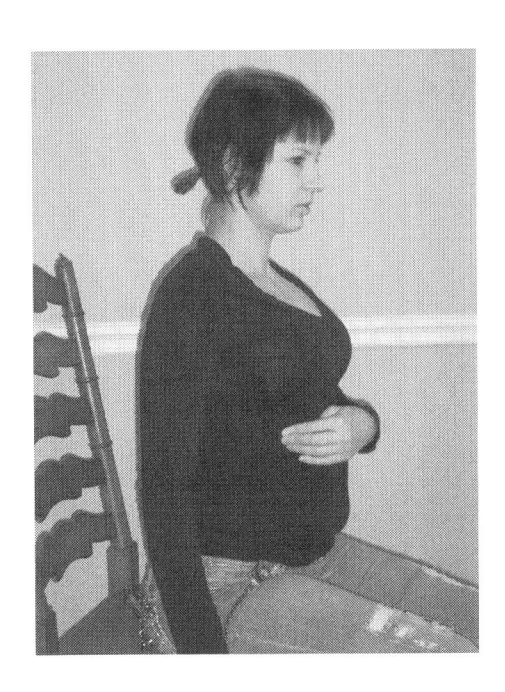

Adjusting Front Rib, Press the Rib as Needed

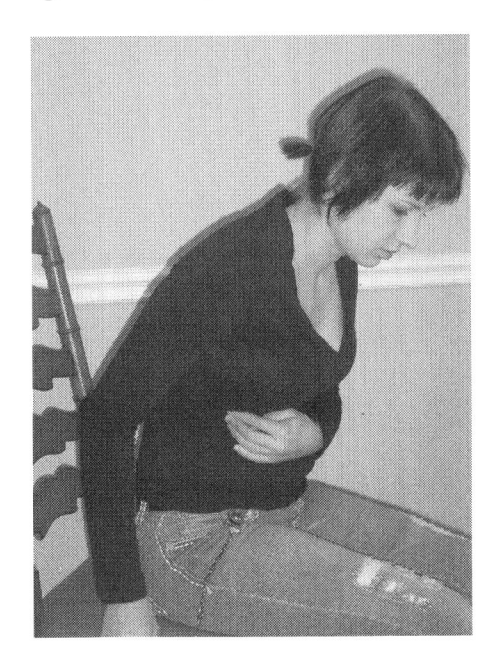

Roll Forward

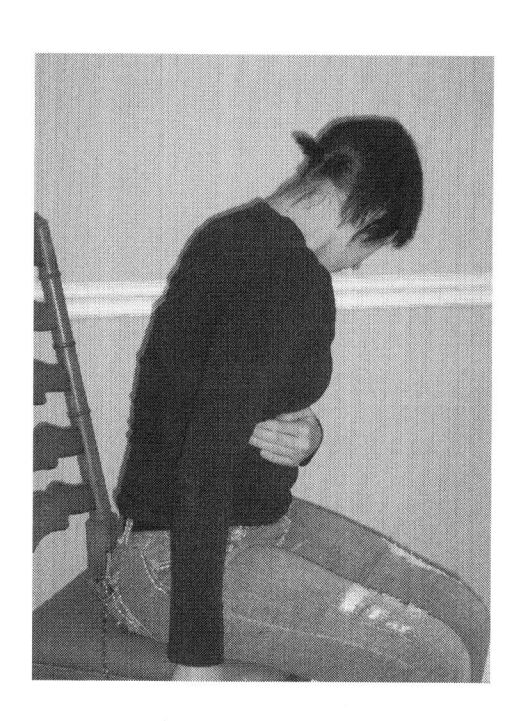

Rotate to the Left

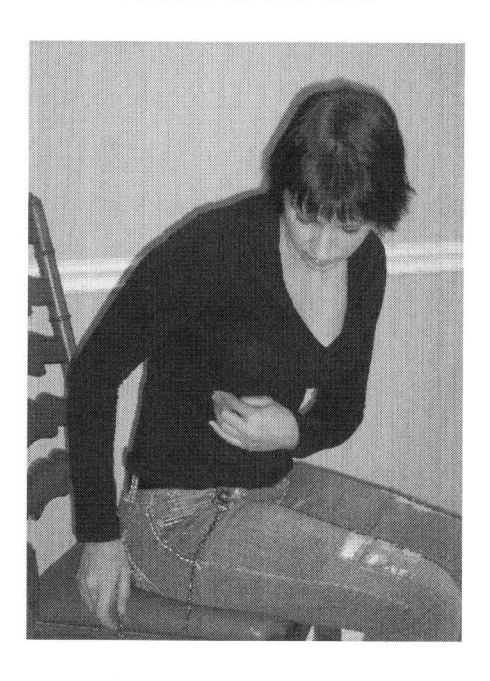

Rotate to the Right

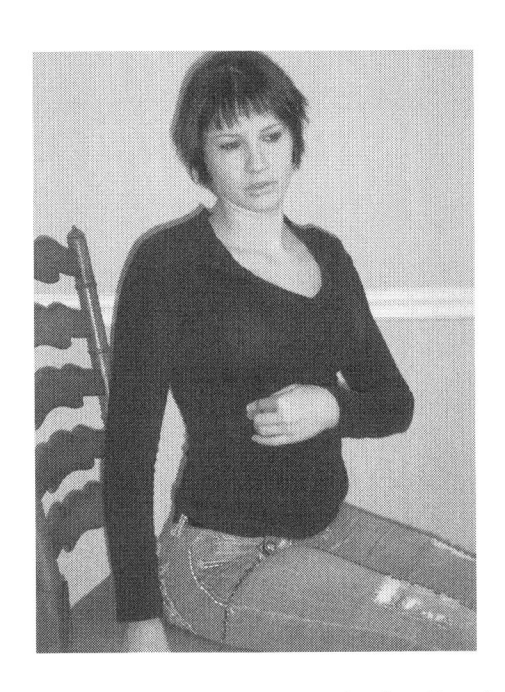

Come Upright and Arch the Back

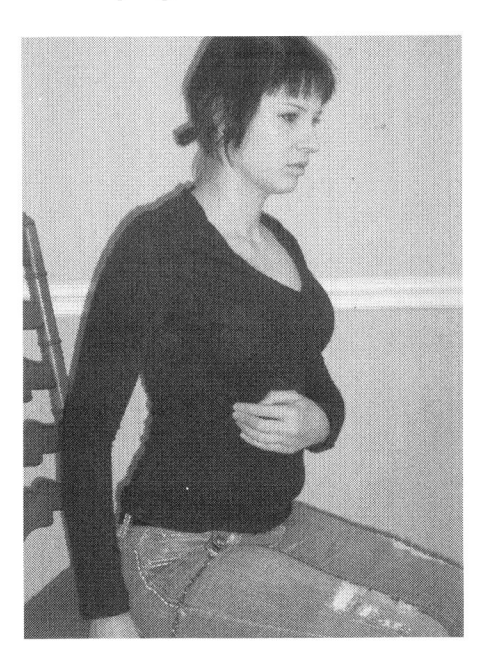

Turn Back Forward Before Releasing the Arch

Adjusting the Top Ribs

This method is new, very effective and easy to do. It is good for adjusting the first three ribs and in many cases the fourth one as well. The biggest limit is how far down you can reach.

The technique is to rotate your arm around as you apply downward pressure on each of the ribs separately.

While pressing down on the top rib with the opposite side hand rotates the free arm forward, up, back and down. Repeat on the next rib down and continue until you do all the upper ribs you can reach.

Next, work up with the adjustment. You can go up and down three or four times for best results though once may be enough.

A little movement in the upper body can help. It only takes a slight twist along with a slight forward to back movement in the torso along with the arm movement.

Practice without the extra torso movement first, that will usually do the trick. As you work with the adjustment you may start to feel how the upper body can naturally move to help with the adjustments.

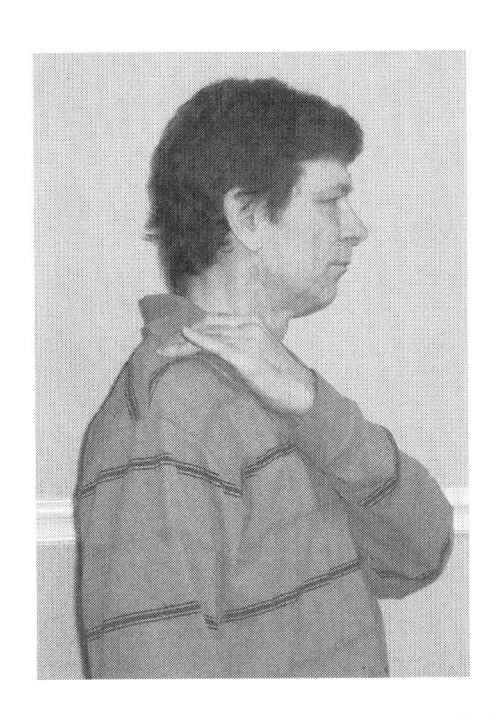

Upper Rib Adjustment, Press the Rib Down

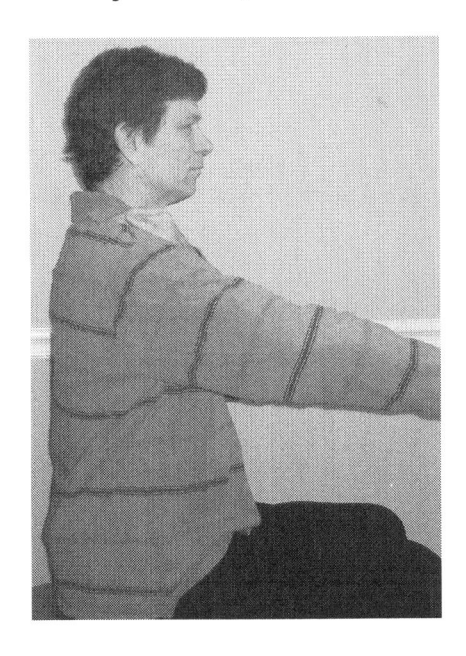

Roll the Shoulder and Arm Forward

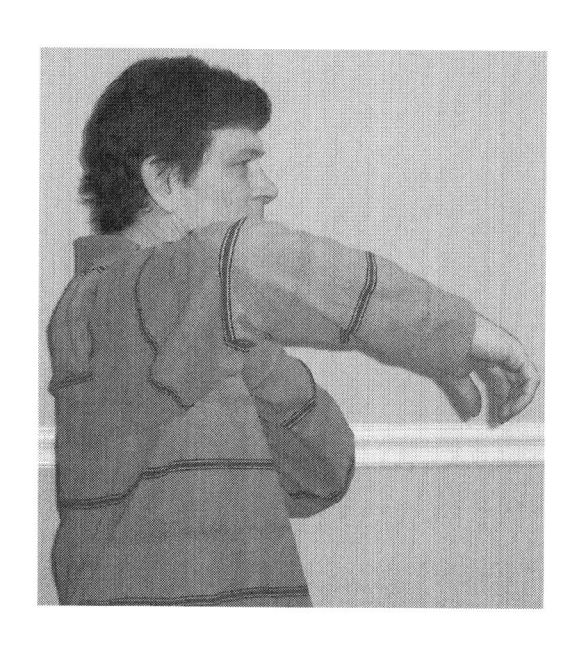

Continue Moving the Shoulder and Arm Up

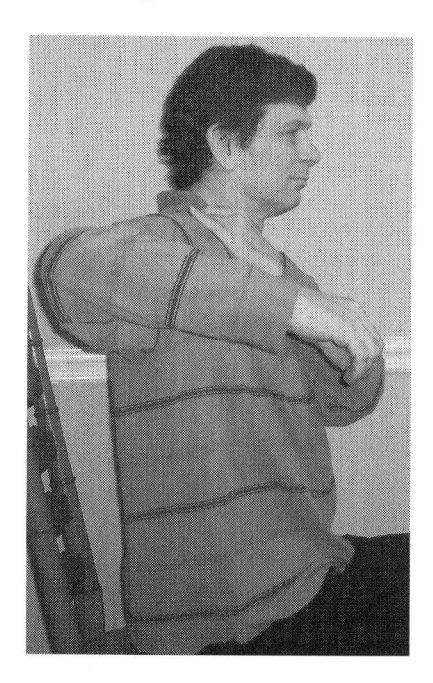

Take the Shoulder and Arm Back and down to the Starting Position

Adjusting Ribs You Can't Reach

You will be able to reach and adjust most of the ribs in the upper and lower back as well as all the ribs in the front. But, it is impossible to reach and press hard enough to adjust the ribs in the middle back. For this you will need help from a friend or a massage tool.

While I recommend a light pressure to adjust the spine, especially in the neck, the ribs can take quite a bit more pressure. Part of the reason you want to apply more pressure is to make sure you maintain contact with the rib as you do the adjustment.

This is more like getting a nice massage than an adjustment. Like getting a massage, more pressure usually just feels better.

On occasion though, the area around misaligned ribs will be very tender to pressure especially if they have been out for a long time. In this case, a lighter touch may be needed, and that usually works just fine. If nothing else, the muscles will probably start to release, and as you adjust the area a second or third time you may be able to apply more pressure.

Be careful to not over work an area that is particularly sore or inflamed as you can aggravate the muscles. It is often better to give the area some time while you relax or even take a hot soak in the tub.

I once had a couple of ribs go out of alignment so severely that I could barely move. I was lying on a friends couch with no one around, and my massage tool way in another room.

I was probably just lying in an awkward position which pushed two or three ribs out of alignment, but any movement really hurt. I could barely breathe it hurt so much that I could barely struggle to a sitting position. I couldn't reach the ribs that were causing the pain, and it seemed impossible to get up to get my massage tool.

I looked around, and there happened to be a maraca within reach. Why not try using the handle to push on the rib for the adjustment? It was awkward, but it worked!

The pain greatly diminished after I got one or two ribs in so I was able to get my massage tool and take care of the other ribs.

The point is that you can probably find or make something to do the job if needed. Massage tools are great though, and I highly recommend them. Besides, it is really great for working those sore and tired muscles in the back, after you have adjusted the ribs and spine.

Many people have fashioned their own massage tool with inexpensive material or even with something they had around the house or workshop. You might like to do the same to save time or money.

One person used two "L" bracket shelf holders screwed together to form an S shaped tool. This worked great for her and cost very little.

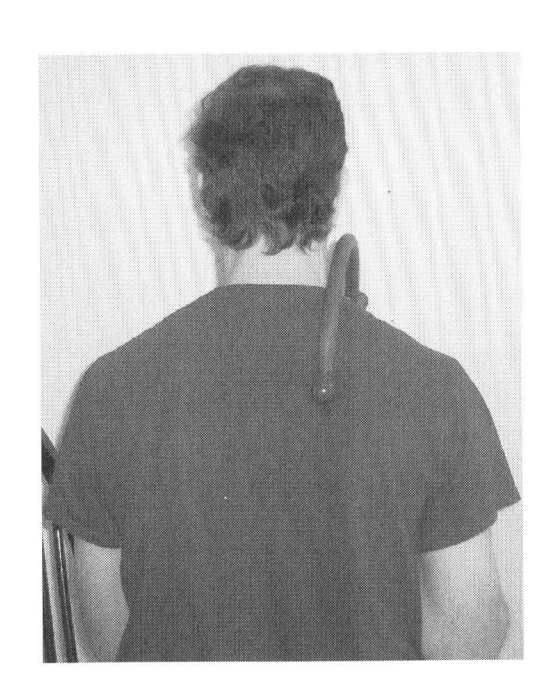

Adjusting Back Ribs with Massage Tool

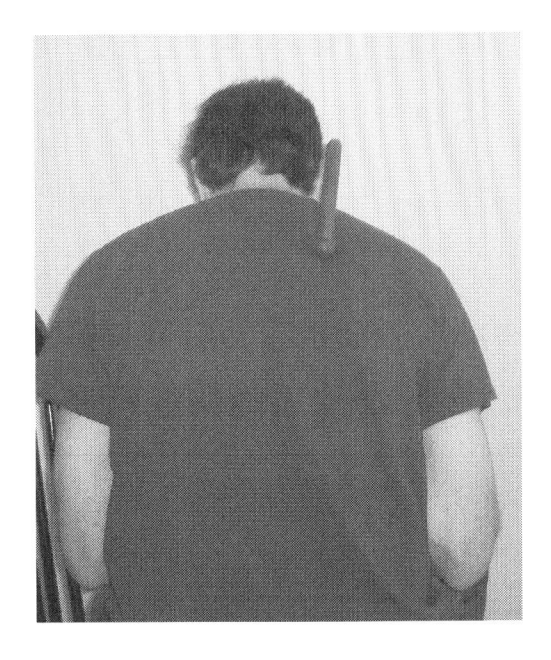

Roll Forward

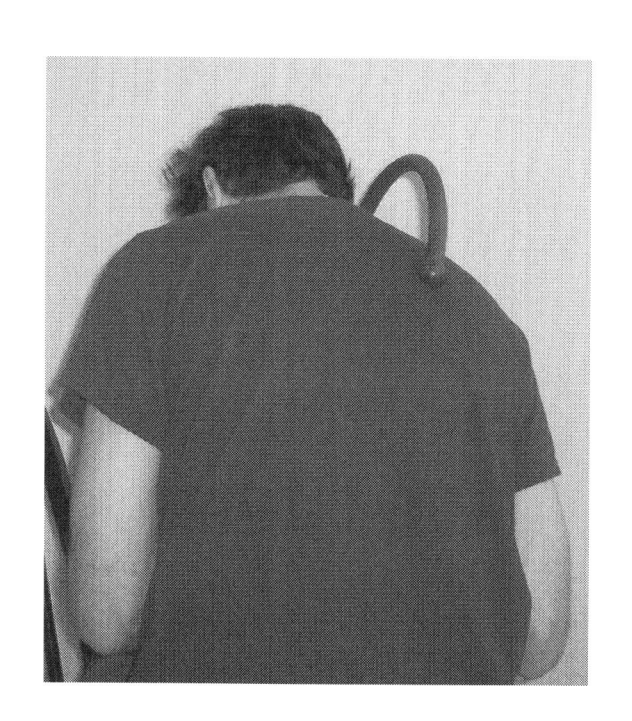

Rotate to the Left

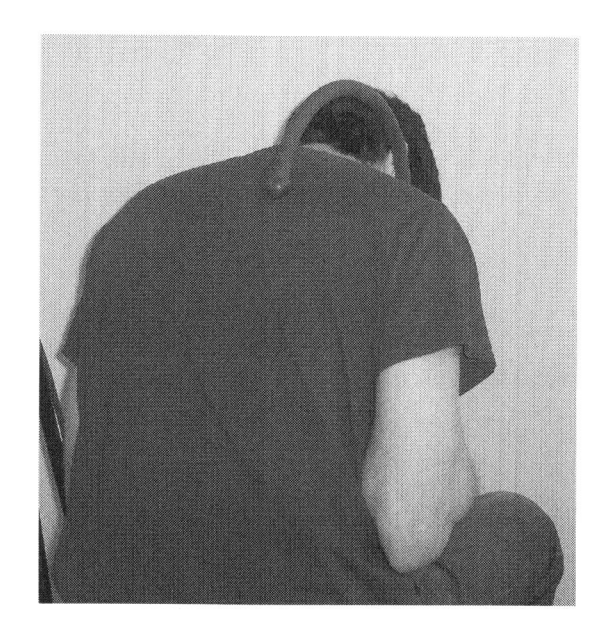

Rotate to the Right

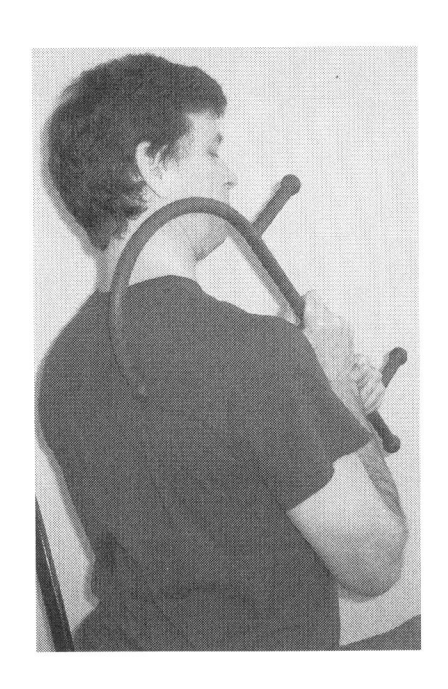

Come Up and Arch the Back

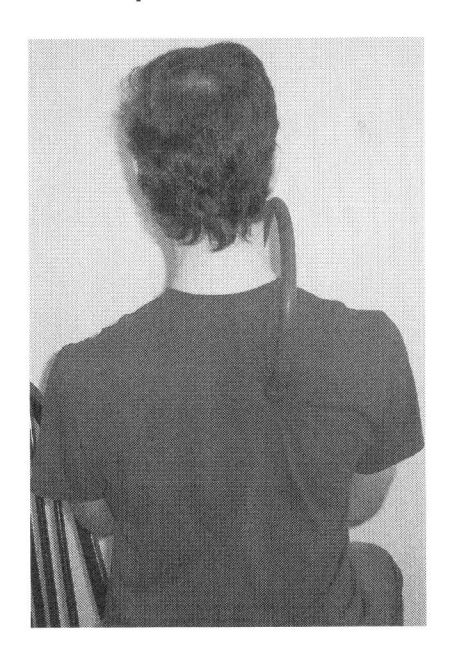

Turn Forward While Still Arched

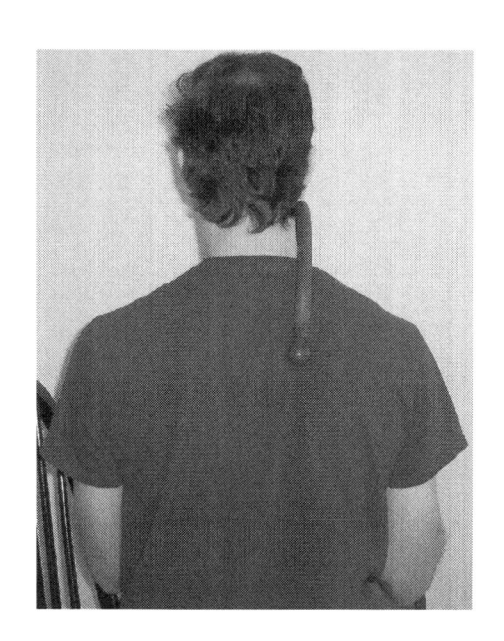

Release

Notes on Adjusting the Ribs

Often the rib will adjust but one or more muscles will still feel sore. Or, there may still be a knot in the muscle. A good way to tell if the rib is back in place is to take a deep breath and see how it feels.

Better yet, take a deep breath or two before adjusting, that way you can tell if it is easier to take a deep breath after the adjustment. Sometimes the deep breath can be painful if the rib is really out. It can even feel like a broken rib.

If you suspect that you have a broken rib from a fall or other injury, it would be a good idea to have an x-ray before attempting to adjust any suspected broken rib. Adjusting a broken rib with any method can definitely cause damage and it will really hurt!

Adjusting the Collar Bone

The collar bones run from just to the side of the hollow at the bottom of the throat to the top of the shoulder toward the front.

Either end of the collar bone can go out of alignment. And, it can go out either up or down.

Find the direction it has moved by finding where it is sore or tender above or below either end. It will be tender on the side it has moved to.

The adjustment is the same for each end of the collar bone. If it needs to move up you push it up from the tender side as you rotate your arm forward, up, back and down. If it needs to move down you press down on it while you rotate the arm back, up, forward and down.

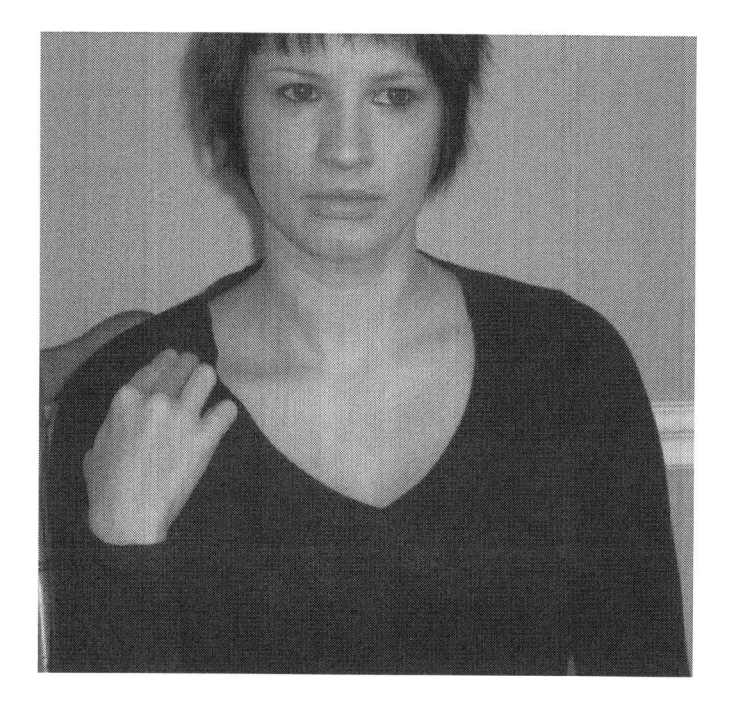

Collar Bone Location near the Shoulder

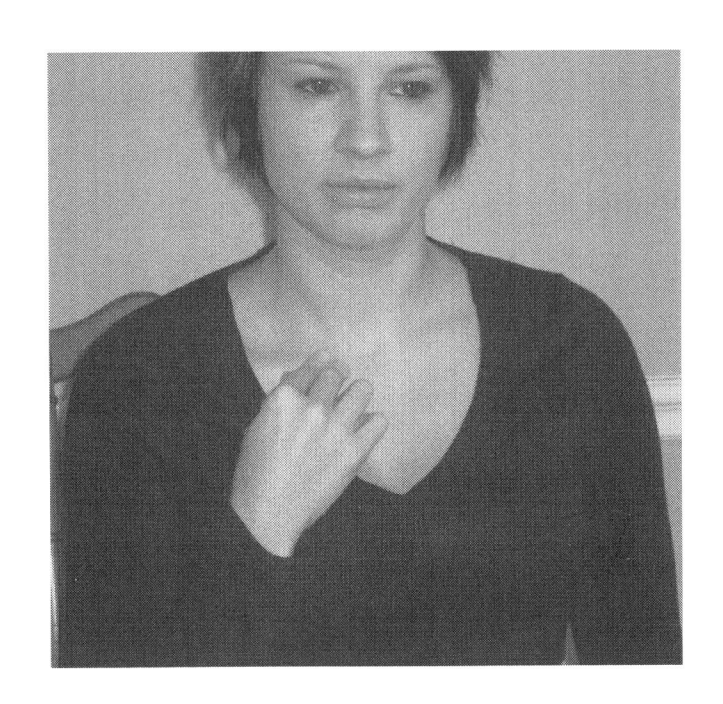

Collar Bone Location near Throat

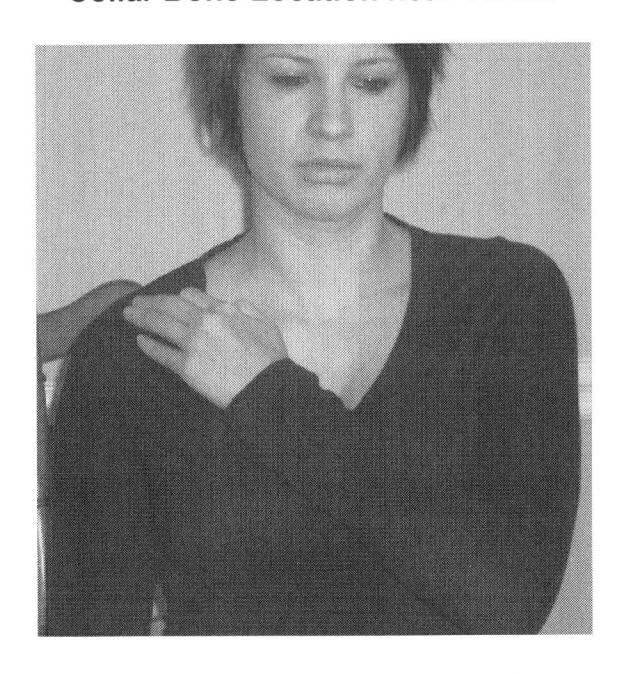

Adjusting Collar Bone Pressing Down

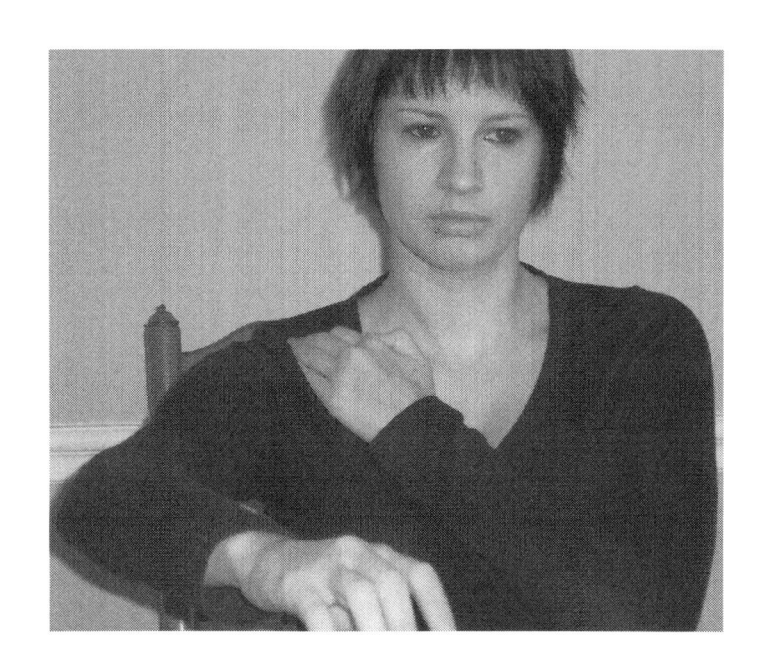

Take the Arm Forward

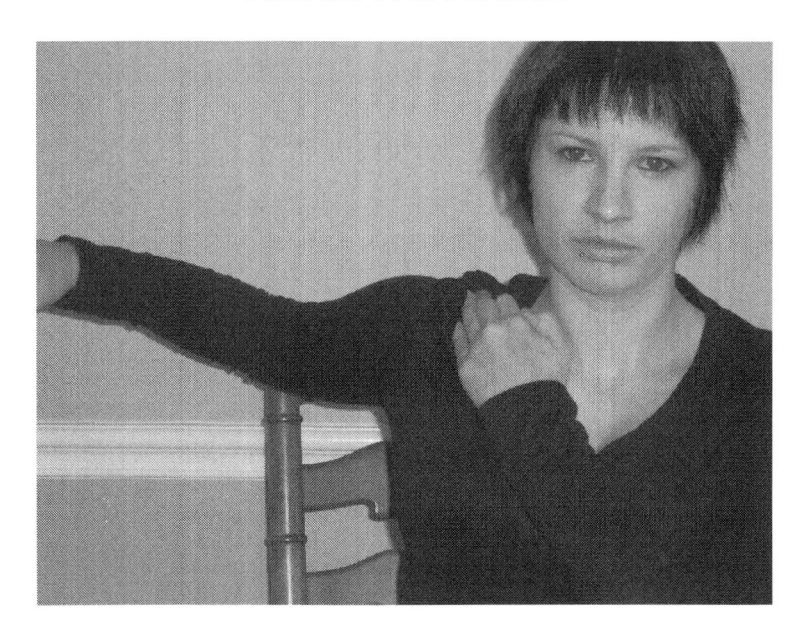

Take the Arm Back

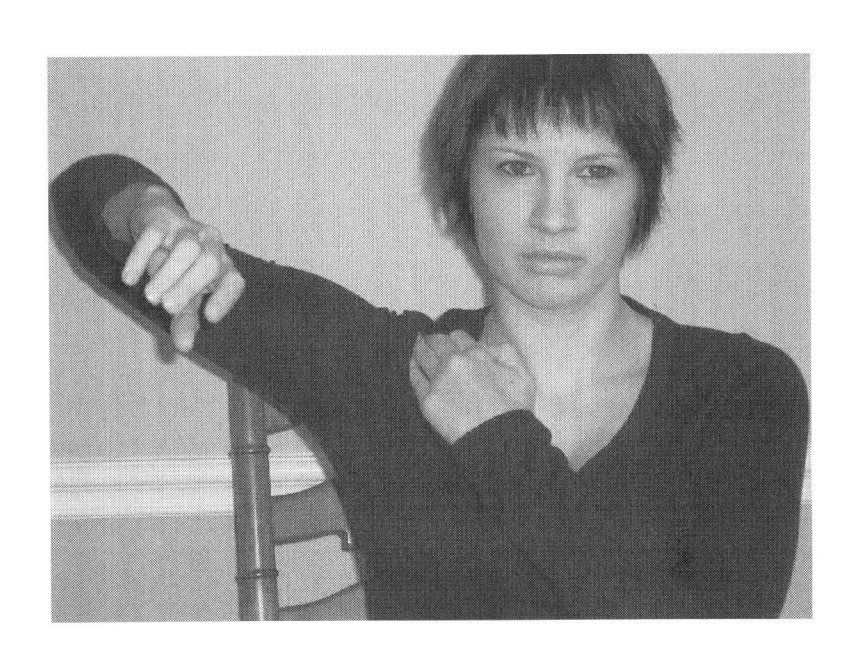

Continue Forward

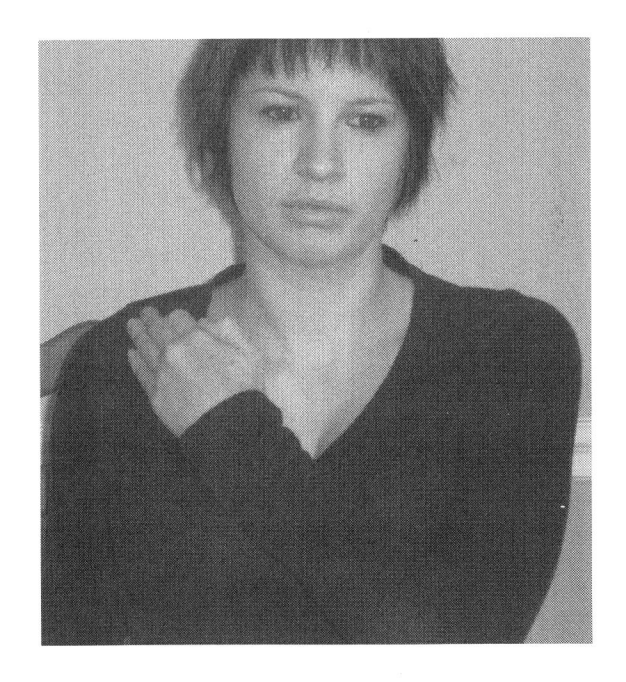

And Back Down to the Beginning Position

The Lower Back

There are many considerations when it comes to the lower back. If you have chronic lower back pain you need to read about the adrenal glands before attempting any adjustment on the sacrum or hips that are discussed in this section.

If you do adjust the hips or sacrum and it is more uncomfortable than before the adjustment then you will know that you need to do something about your adrenal glands. The stretches for the lower back below can give you some relief until the adrenal glands are strong and healthy again.

Another major consideration with the lower back is if there is a disk issue.

A relatively minor disk issue is a bulging disk. Medical science considers this a major issue; however a bulging disk can usually be healed in a six to twelve weeks using natural techniques.

A herniated disk is another thing altogether. In many cases surgery may be called for. No adjustment of any kind should ever be done directly on a herniated disk. It will only cause pain and possibly more problems.

However, adjustments can usually be made when there is a bulging disk as long as it is relatively minor.

Bulging and herniated disks in the lower back are almost always caused by issues that have to do with the adrenal glands. And, they almost always happen between L5 and the sacrum.

This has to do with the fact that when the adrenal glands

and their relationship with the pituitary and hypothalamus glands is out of balance the abdominal muscles will weaken. Without abdominal strength there is no support for the lower back and the disk will bulge as the spine compresses.

This imbalance has to do with excess consumption of sugar and other processed food. This is discussed in detail in the section on the adrenal glands.

Another connection is that the adrenal glands use a lot of the same nutrients as ligaments and tendons. Since the lower back supports the entire weight of the upper body those ligaments and tendons tend to weaken sooner than others. Of course, there are exceptions.

My daughter, when she was doing a lot of gymnastics, had ligament problems first show up in her wrists from doing hand stands. Treating her adrenal glands ended that problem almost immediately.

Stretching the Lower Back

Be aware if there is any pain at all when doing any stretch, and stop if it hurts. Also, it is a good idea to come out of a stretch like these after a short time just to check in to see how your body is doing, especially if you are not familiar with the stretch.

The first stretch is a simple twist that may help the lower back, especially if you relax into the position for one to five minutes. The same cautions apply to the second stretch which is a great assisted stretch. I have never seen the assisted stretch cause anything but great relief for lower back pain.

Lower Back Twist Stretch

Start in a reclining position face up. Draw your right knee into your chest and take it across your body to the left side. Take the knee all the way to the floor if you can. You will need to shift your hips around to get into a comfortable position so that you can relax into the twist.

Draw your left leg slightly up toward your body. You can place your left hand on your right knee to help counter balance so that you can completely relax into the stretch.

Reach your right hand and arm out to the right side. In the full twist your right shoulder blade will be off the floor.

If your right shoulder is uncomfortable you can place your right hand on the ribcage on the right side allowing your elbow and shoulder to release toward the floor.

As you breathe your right shoulder will rise and fall helping to take you deeper into the twist with each exhale. Relax and allow the breath to carry you deeper into the stretch.

Alternate
Try this method if you are having trouble getting into this position so that you can relax into the twist. Start in a side lying position on your left side. Adjust your legs so that you are comfortable with the left leg extended a little more than the right.

Next, take your right hand over to the right side opening your position up into the twist. Adjust your position as above.

You can have the lower leg more extended or draw the legs up further as shown in the photos below.

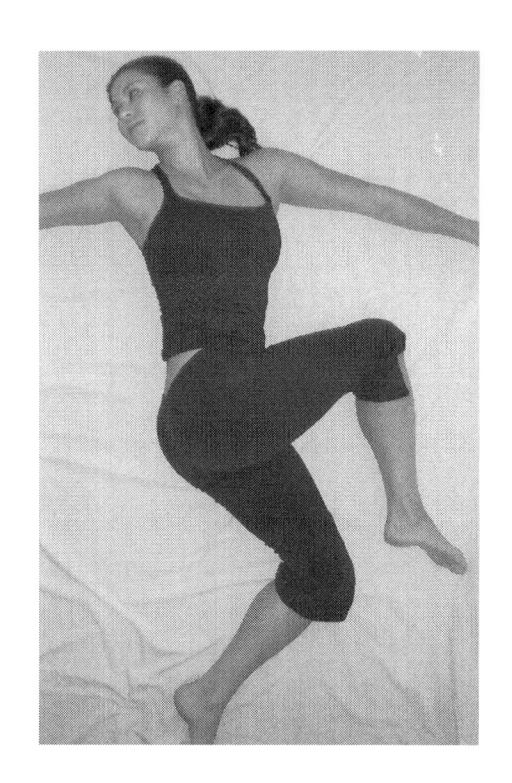

Reclining Twist

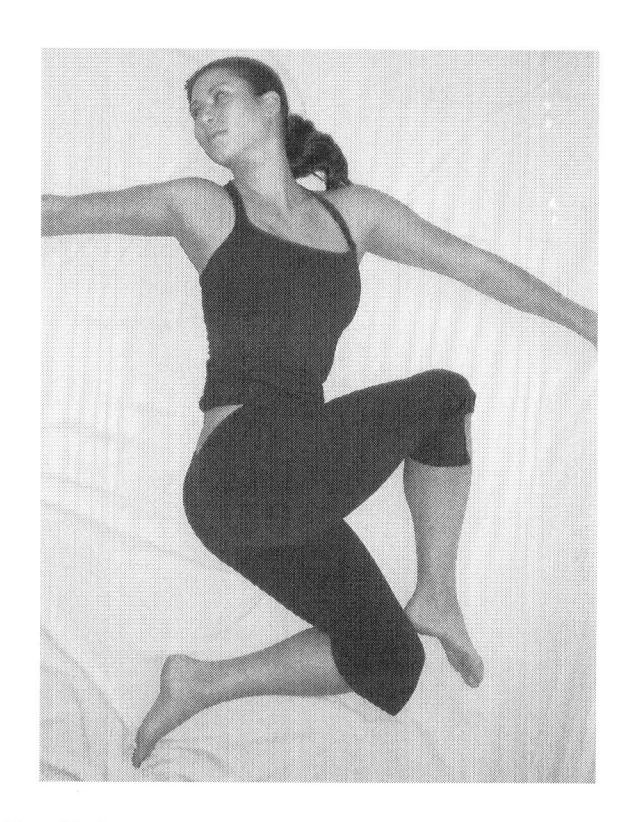

Reclining Twist Knees Drawn Up Variation

Deeper Reclining Twist

This is a similar twist that is deeper that many people like.

Start by lying down on your back with your knees bent up so the soles of the feet are on floor. Cross your right leg over the left so the knees are close to each other. Some people like to hook the right foot behind the left leg, but this doesn't work for everyone and it is not necessary.

Take your legs over to the left side, ideally until the right knee is touching the ground. In this position, your left leg would be on top of the right which would help you into the stretch.

You may find an even deeper stretch if you draw your legs closer in toward your body.

Reach your right hand and arm to the right side as above. Put your right hand on the rib cage if the right shoulder is uncomfortable reaching straight out.

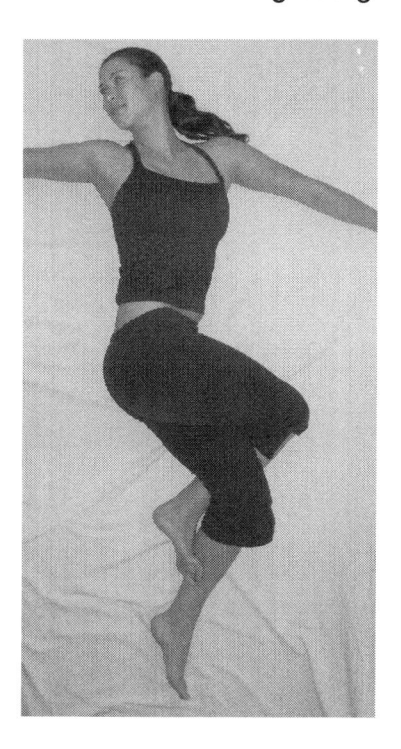

Reclining Deep Twist Legs Wrapped

Lower Back Assisted Ligament Stretch

Ideally you would have a friend help you with this stretch. But, some people will be able to do it on themselves. Give it a try and see how it works for you.

Start by lying on your back. Draw your knees toward your chest and take them over to the right side. You would be lying in a twist similar to the one described above but with the legs together.

Your helper places their right palm on your lower back and their left hand on your knees. They then press the knees in toward your body and up toward your head. The right hand presses into the lower back and pulls down away from your head.

It is like a spiral movement, but of course there is little motion, except to draw you into the stretch.

Have them hold you in this stretch for several seconds, up to a half a minute. Relax into the stretch, it should feel really good.

You can have them help you into this stretch again if you like, but come out to check in to see how your body is doing. Of course, stop if there is any pain at all. Repeat on the other side.

If doing it yourself you would use your right hand or arm to pull your knees in and up while pressing down and away with your left hand.

The more pressure you apply the better. At least up to a point though, a very strong helper could go too far.

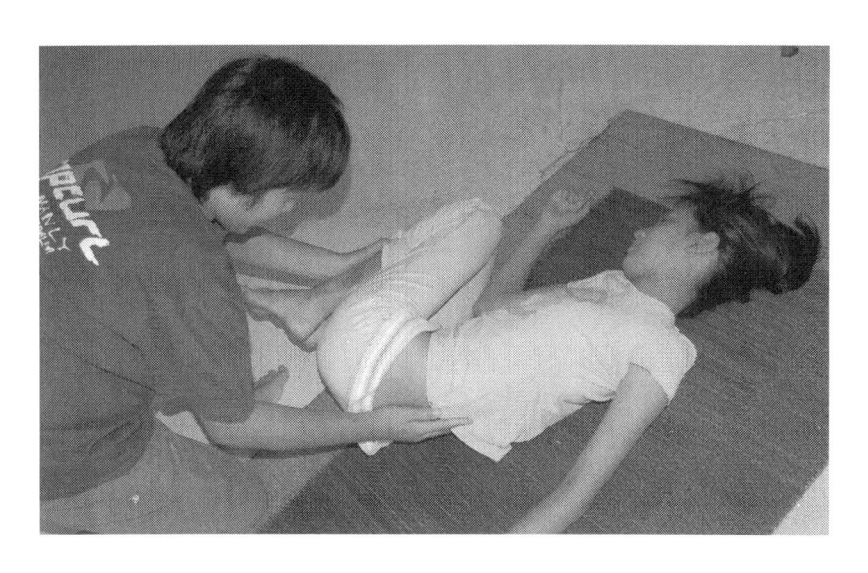

**Assisted Ligament Stretch
Press Down on the Lower Back and
Press the Knees in and Up**

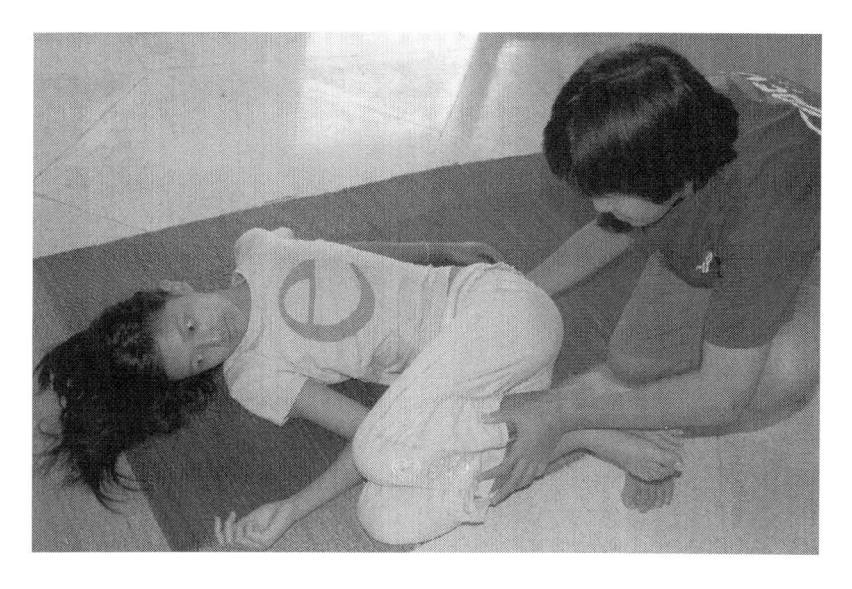

Ligament Stretch Alternate View

The Sacrum

The sacrum is a triangular bone made up of five fused vertebra. Most lower back pain involves the sacrum and where it connects with the hip bone. However, sometimes the sacrum will be all that is out of alignment especially if the discomfort is minor. If it is very uncomfortable or painful, then most likely both the sacrum and where it connects with the hips will both be out of alignment.

What a Sacral Misalignment Is

The sacrum is at the very lower back in between the hips. It almost always goes out of alignment by tilting under.

To get a picture of this, place your hand on your sacrum. The hand is longer than the sacrum, so most of the palm will be on the top with your fingers at the bottom and below. Tilt your hand so the fingers start to reach down and under the tailbone, the palm will drop down and slightly away from where it is touching. This is the most common direction the sacrum will tilt out of alignment. The adjustment direction is obvious and discussed below.

The other direction is incredibly rare. The only time I find this is when doing sensitive craniosacral work, and that misalignment is very subtle. I have never seen a sacrum that is tilted up cause discomfort though I have heard of it.

Using the same hand position as above, take the heel of your hand up and imagine it moving into your back while the fingers move away from where they are touching.

That is the opposite or uncommon shift that the sacrum can move out of alignment.

Sacral Adjustment Reclining Twist

I recommend that you adjust the sacrum on both sides even if you feel relief after doing one side. You may not actually need to do the second side, however both sides usually need the adjustment.

You can do this adjustment on any surface. A firm surface such as the floor with carpeting or a light mat works well, or you can do it while lying on a bed or futon. We'll take it from lying on the floor.

Unlike the previous Self Adjusting Techniques, this method does require some pressure, and therefore some strength, to work well, though it can work with only a little pressure.

We'll start with adjusting the sacrum on the right side.

Start by lying on your back with your legs together or close together. This is the starting and ending position. Draw your right knee in toward your chest and take the leg to the left across your body so that the right knee is near or on the floor. Shift your hip around so that you are fully in the twist. Place the heel of your right hand on your sacrum so that you can apply some pressure, and the heel of the left hand on the right ASIS or hip point in the front.

The left hand isn't really needed, but it is a nice assistance to help guide the hips around. In these photos she isn't using her left hand; you can see an example of that in the photos for the reclining SI twist technique below.

The main adjustment comes from the right hand directly on the sacrum pulling up. Strength is needed to press into the sacrum so that you can keep the hand firmly in contact with the sacrum. You are actually moving the sacrum, so the main action is to pull up on it. The left hand can press against the ASIS for a counter to the pressure of the right hand.

As you pull up on the sacrum, extend your right leg and roll onto your back. Continue on around with your body and the right leg until you are completely flat with your leg back on the floor next to or near the left leg. This isn't a fast movement. Take your time so the bones can move gently. Take maybe three or four seconds to come completely around. Repeat on the other side.

This adjustment won't work for everyone because of physical limitations. Some people may not be able to reach the back well enough, or they may not have enough strength. This can also be difficult for pregnant women. The walking method works really well. I include this method to give you an alternate, and because sometimes the back really hurts. If you are already lying down you can just adjust it before trying to get up.

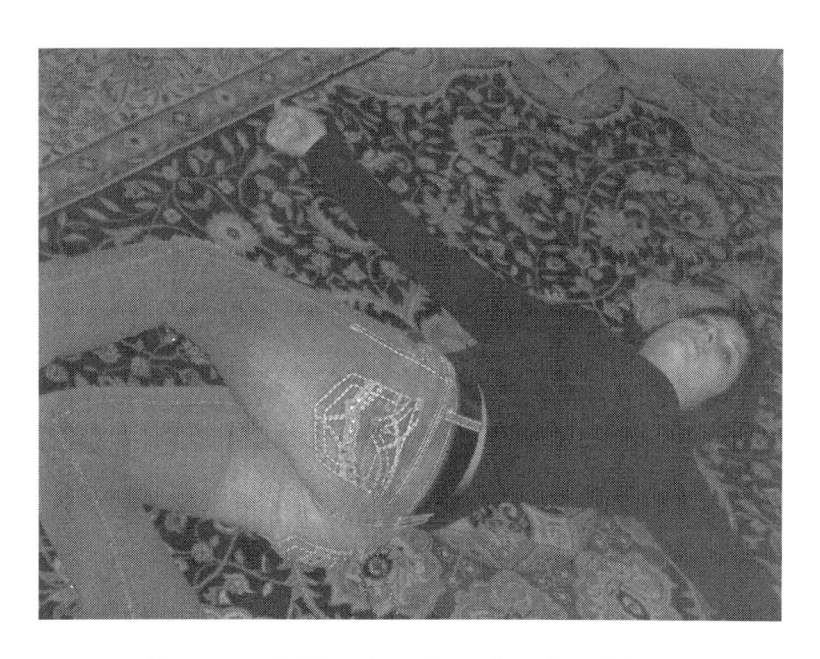

Sacrum Adjusting Starting Position

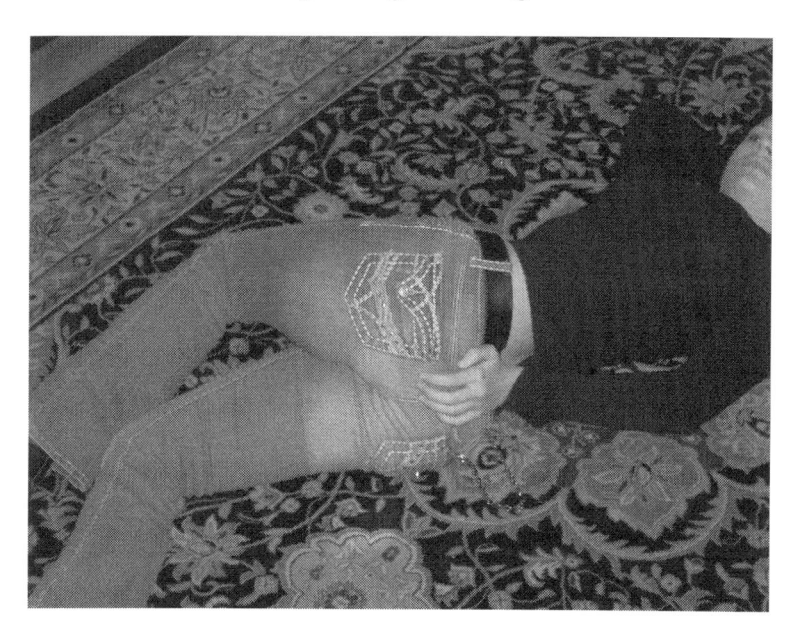

Pull the Sacrum Up with the Heel of the Hand

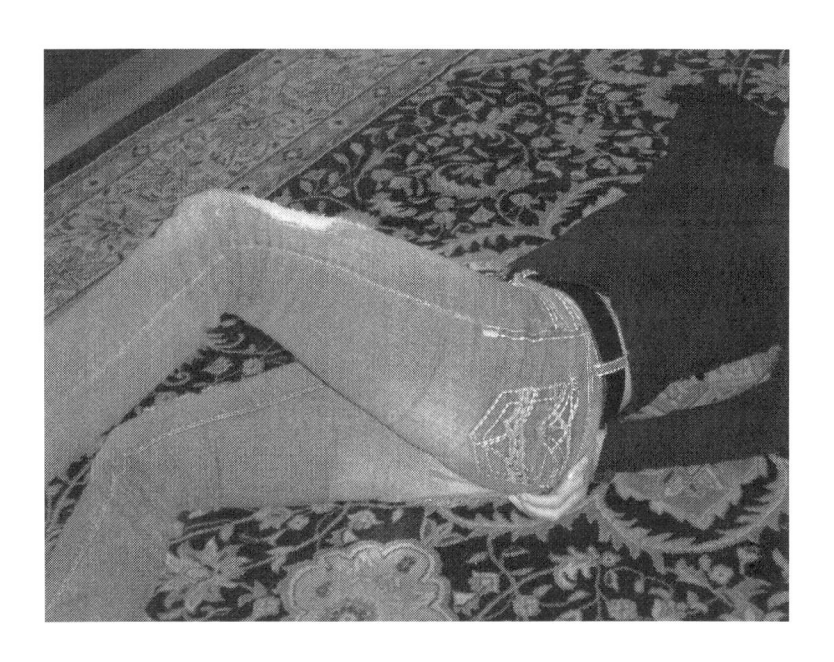

Bring the Top Leg Up

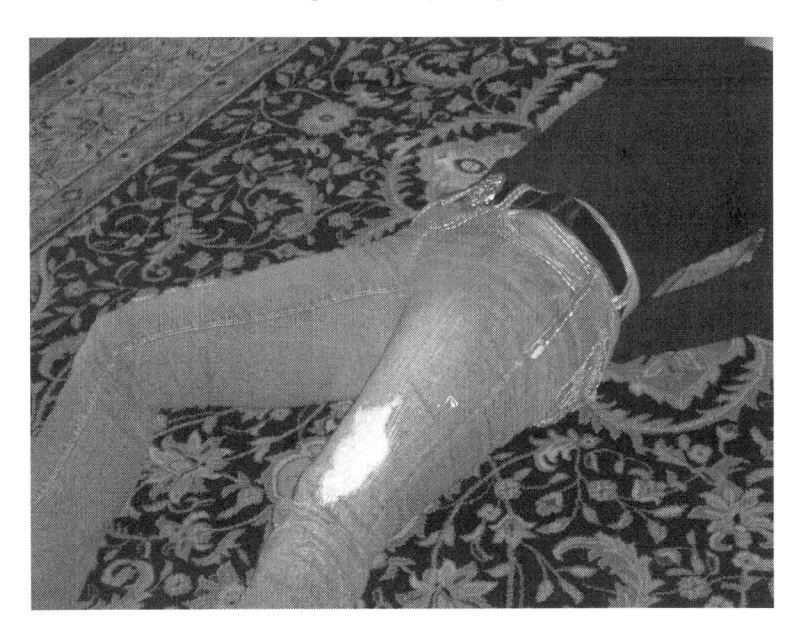

Bring the Top Leg to the Floor

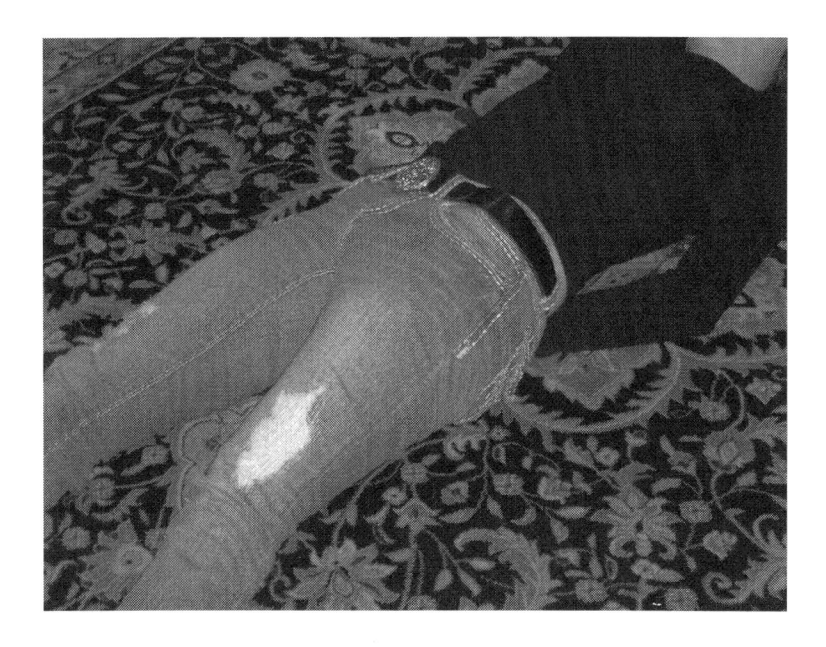

And Along Side the Bottom Leg, Straighten Both

Sacrum Walking Adjustment

The other way to adjust the sacrum is very easy if you are able to reach the sacrum. You also need to be strong enough to pull up on it while walking. That's really all there is to it.

Use the heel of your right hand to pull up on the right side of the sacrum while walking. Lengthen through your back as you walk. Repeat while pulling up on the other side.

All the walking techniques only need three to eight steps to affect the adjustment. On occasion more may be needed though.

Some people can do this adjustment with the fingers, but most won't have the strength to press in and pull up enough to affect the adjustment.

If you can't easily reach the sacrum, or lack the strength to pull up on it you can use a massage tool.

This is the first way I figured out how to adjust the sacrum and most of the joints in my back and hips. I later developed the reclining method because at times my back hurt too much for me to even get out of bed! This is when I was in really bad shape. I still like the reclining method because it is easy, and I don't have to get up to feel better. I have even gotten so that I can do the same action while standing. I just lean against a wall or other solid structure and do the same action as the reclining method.

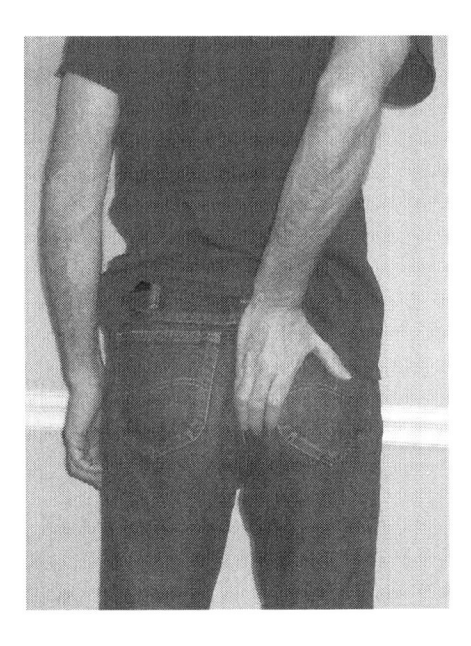

Place the Heel of the Hand on the Sacrum

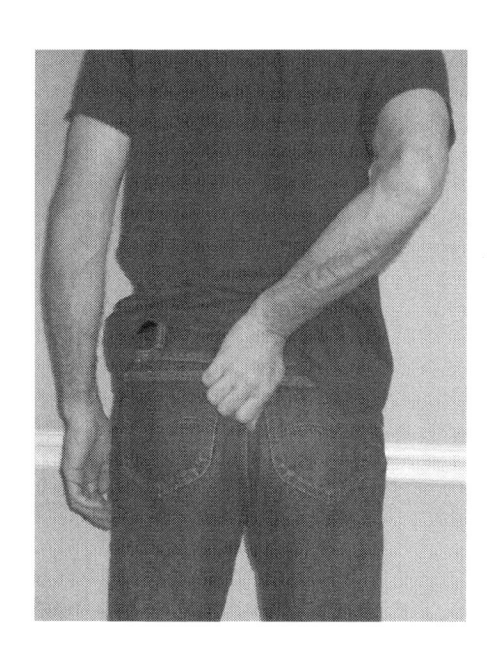

Or Use the Base of the Thumb

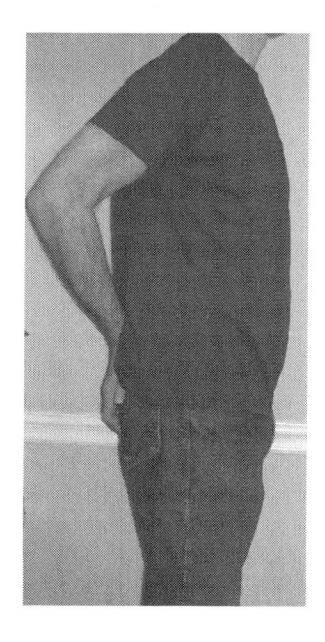

Pull Up on the Sacrum

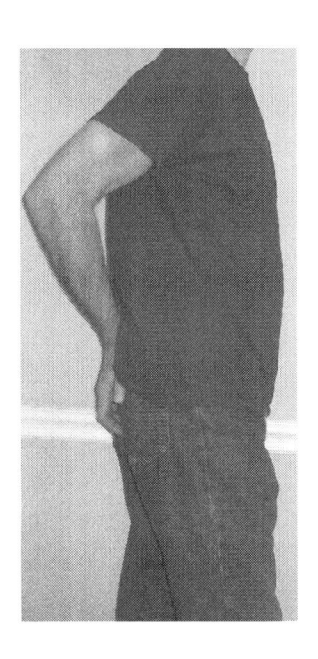

Continue Pulling Up on the Sacrum as You Walk

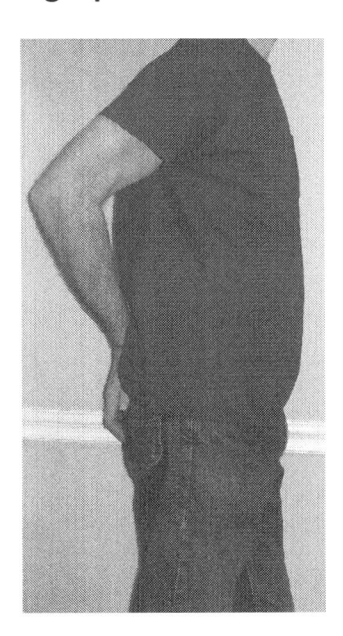

Walk for a Few Steps to Adjust

Using a massage tool to pull on the sacrum is a lot easier than using your hand. Use the massage tool to push in and pull up on the top of the sacrum.

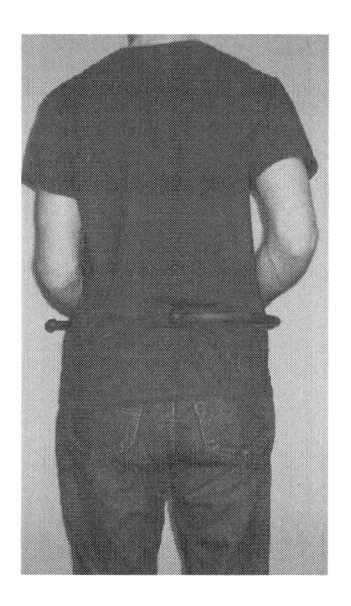

Hook the Massage Tool on the Sacrum

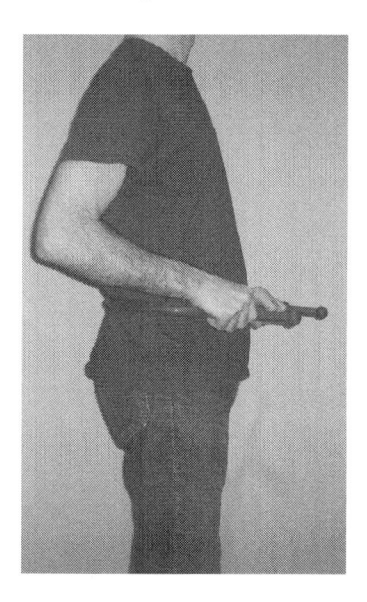

Pull the Massage Tool, Lengthen Through the Spine

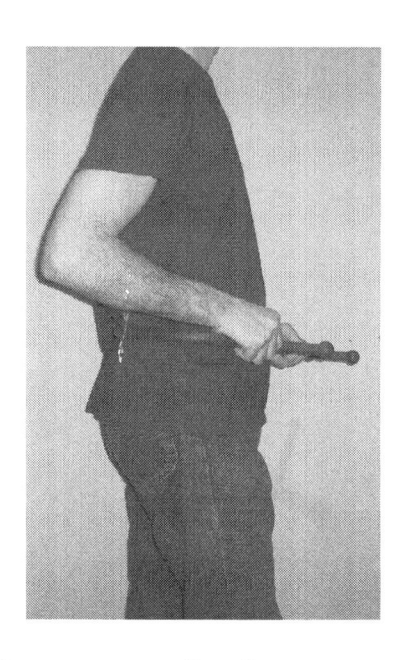

Keep Pressure on the Sacrum and Walk

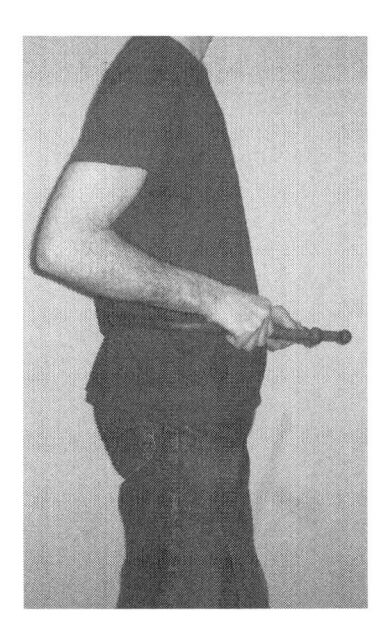

Keep Your Spine Tall as You Take Several Steps

The Hips and Sacroiliac Joint

Physiology of Hip Misalignments

The triangular shaped sacrum sets down into the hip structure in the back. This is where the weight of the upper body is transferred into the hips and from there into the legs.

The hips are a solid structure with the prominent hip bones in the front, the ASIS bones. Approximately opposite to the ASIS bones are the PSIS bones, the prominent hip bones in the back. (See the photo on page 98.) These two sets of bones are the front and back of the top of the hip structure. At the bottom are the sit bones or the ischium. These structures are connected, so any adjustment to the hip structure is going to involve adjusting all the parts.

The way the hip shifts out of alignment can vary, but there is a usual direction. Think of a body from the side facing to your right. Imagine that the hip structure might shift slightly in clockwise or counter clockwise rotation from your point of view. The counter clockwise direction is the most common way the hip goes out of alignment. That is, the PSIS and the sit bones have shifted down, and the ASIS has shifted upward. The adjustment is to move the hip structure in the clockwise direction.

Where the sacrum joins with the hip in the back is called the sacroiliac or SI joint. That is where the sacrum and hips shift causing a misalignment. Usually both shift, but the hip misalignment is the one that tends to cause the most discomfort.

This area is greatly affected by the energy systems discussed in the section on the adrenal glands. As mentioned before, adjusting the SI joint can bring more discomfort or pain if these systems are out of balance. It is worth repeating that if you do this adjustment and your back hurts more then you definitely need to do something to take care of your adrenal glands to insure that your lower back pain will be eliminated. It usually takes only one to three weeks for the program to work so that you can do this adjustment successfully.

How to Know Which Direction the SI is out

The lower back can really hurt when the SI is out of alignment. This is the most common misalignment complaint I see.

People with this condition often move about to try to relieve the discomfort. They twist around, arch the back and round the back. Rounding the back is what usually gives the most relief. If this is the case the SI joint is probably out in the most common direction as mentioned above.

This is how my back was out when I had to always have my knees supported when lying on my back. Several ways to do the adjustment for this common direction are given here. If the back feels better when the back is arched, then the SI is out in the less common direction.

It is interesting to note that sitting will often put the SI out of alignment again. For some people a lumbar pillow, which helps keep the lower back arched, will help.

Sacroiliac Adjustment Reclining Twist

This technique is basically the same as the reclining sacrum adjustment. The only differences are the placement of the hands. Both hands will be actively used in adjusting the SI joint. We'll start with adjusting the left SI joint.

Lie on your back with your legs extended and together. This is the starting and ending position for this adjustment.

Draw your left knee in toward your chest and take it over to the right side. Shift your hips around so you can get fully into the twist.

Use your left hand on your left SI joint and your right hand on your left hip bone in front. As you straighten your left leg you will press the front hip bone down towards your feet and pull your SI joint in front up towards your head.

Follow along with your hands continuing to pull and push the hip as you bring your left leg all the way straight and next to or near your right leg. You will need to squeeze the two hands toward each other so you can apply enough pressure to pull the hip structure into alignment.

Remember the direction that you want the hip to move as described when looking at a body from the side. You want to rotate the hip structure so the back part is moving up while the front part is moving down.

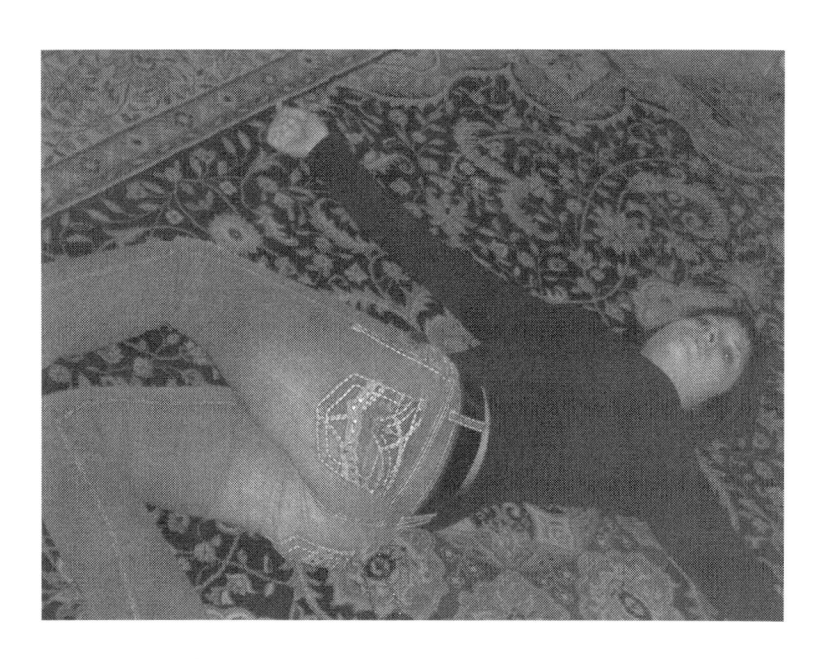

Start in a Deep Reclining Twist

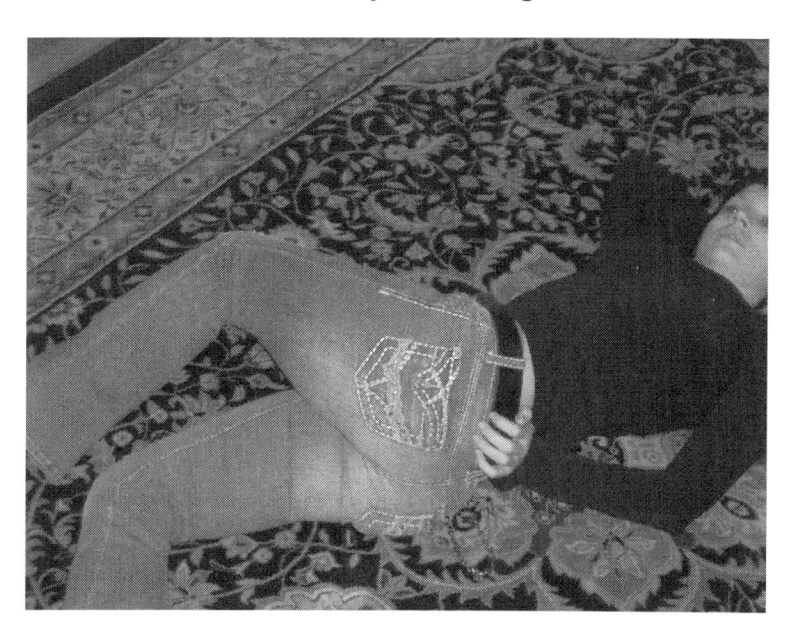

Hold the Front and Back Hip Bones Tightly

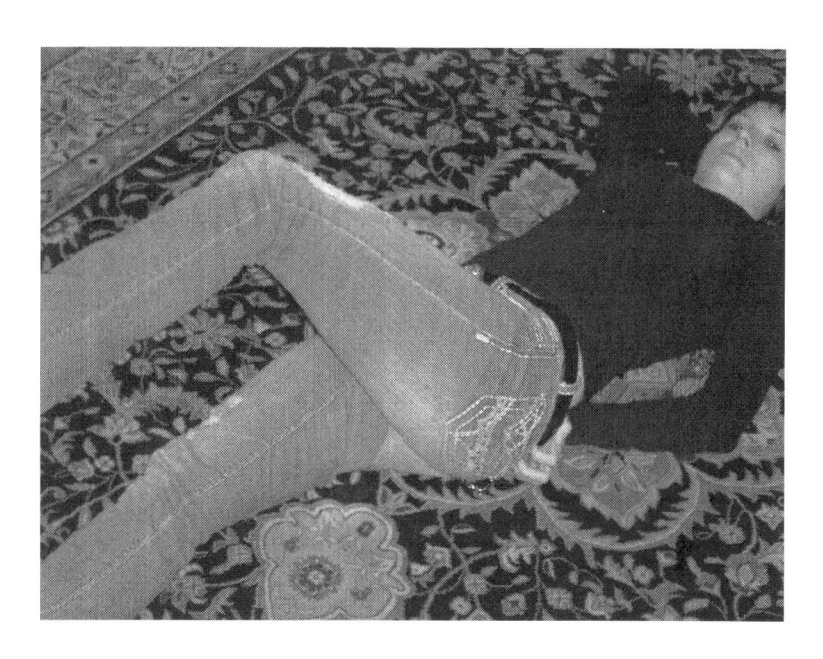

Bring the Top Leg Up While Pulling the Back Hand Up and Pushing Down on the Upper Hand

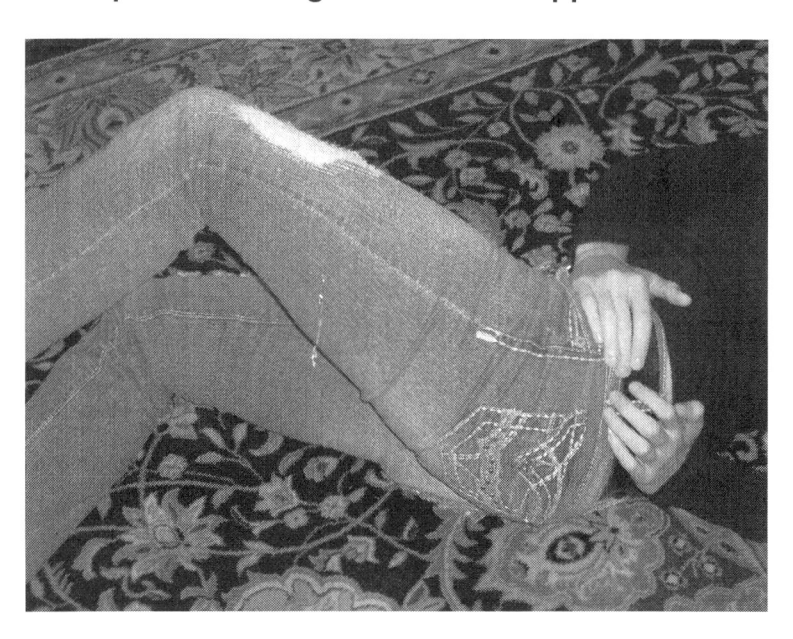

Continue To Push and Pull the Hip Bones While Bringing the Top Leg Up

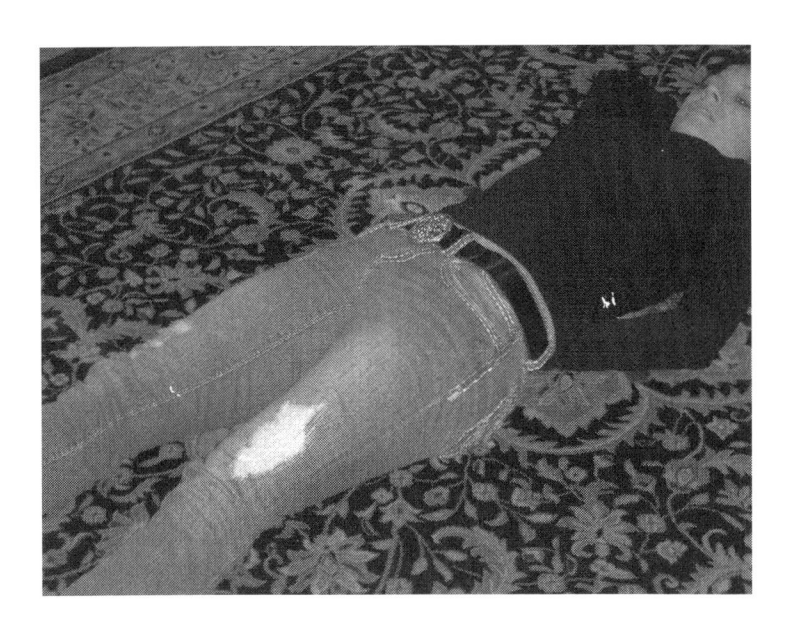

Bring the Top Leg to the Floor While Still Pulling the Back Hip Bone Up

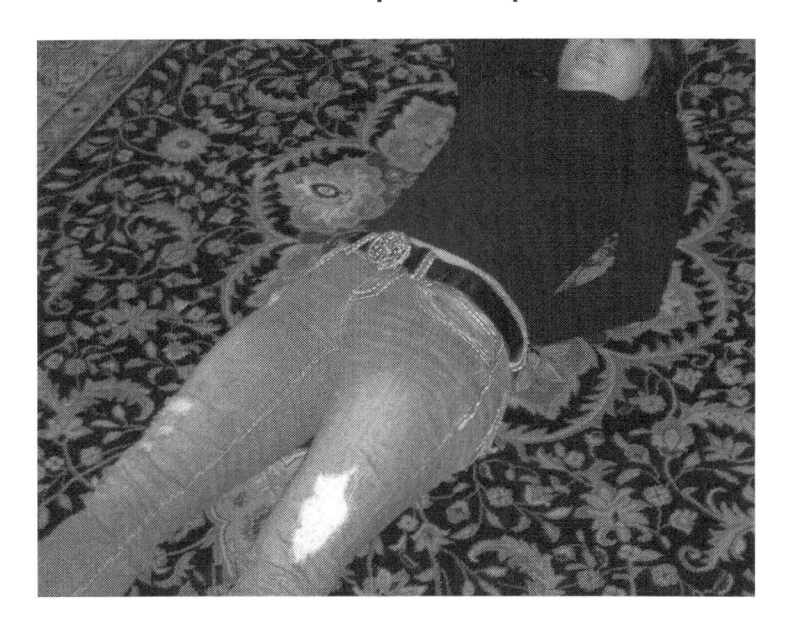

Continue with the Leg taking it Along Side the Bottom Leg, Straighten Both

SI Reclining Blocking Adjustment

Blocking is a method of adjusting that uses support in one area so that another area can release down. Foam triangular blocks are inexpensive and work as well as the expensive models that chiropractors use. However, you can simply use a shoe. Any shoe will work, but a tennis shoe works the best. A pillow rolled up towel or anything that gives the right kind of support will work as well.

Blocking requires a firm surface such as a carpeted floor or a firm mat. Soft surfaces like a bed don't work very well as you cannot get the required lift.

Relief should come right away if the blocking is done right and it is the right adjustment. There may be a little discomfort as you settle into the support, but that should turn to relief very quickly. It usually feels good because the bones are able to settle back into place. Stop right away if it doesn't feel good or if there is pain. Relax into the support for best results.

To block the SI joint insert the shoe or foam wedge under your PSIS (the hip bone in the back) in such a way that the toe is more under C4 and 5, but with a firm lift under the PSIS. Lie on the block for two or three minutes.

You can also do this with your fist on edge so the area around the forefinger and thumb are under the PSIS. The only problem with this is that it can be a little hard on your hand. Repeat on the other side.

The location of PSIS will vary by the size of the person and the width of the hips. You can see the bone on the left side while the right side is pointed to in the photo

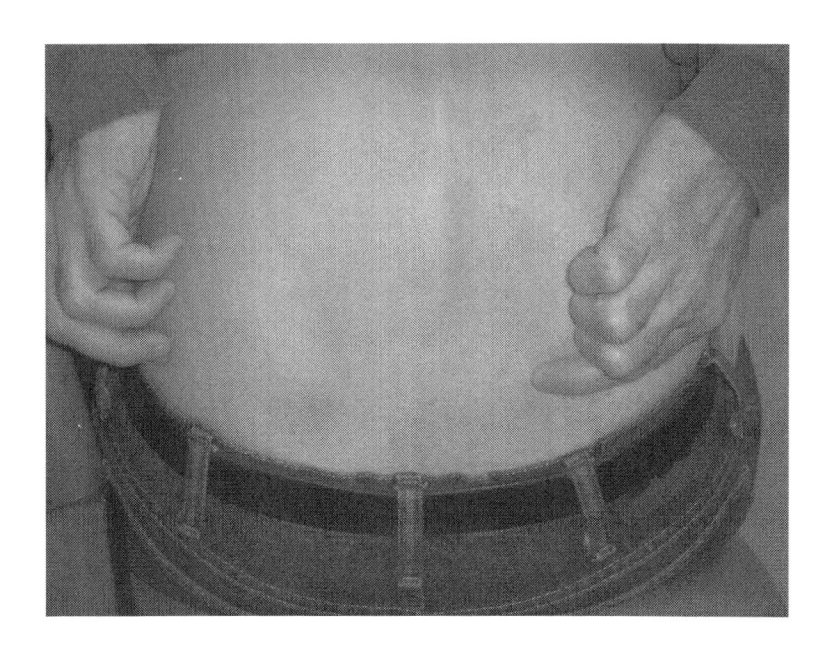

PSIS Location

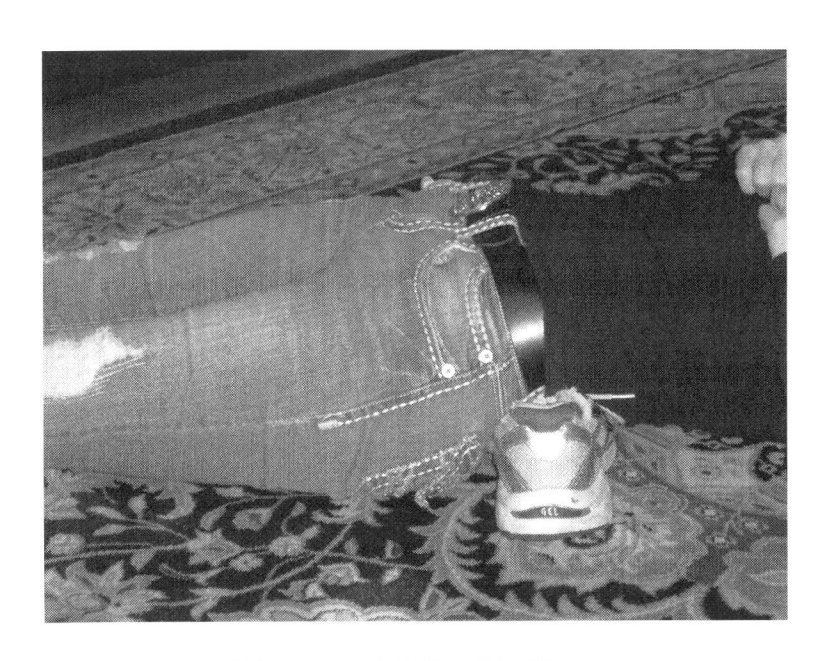

Blocking PSIS with Shoe

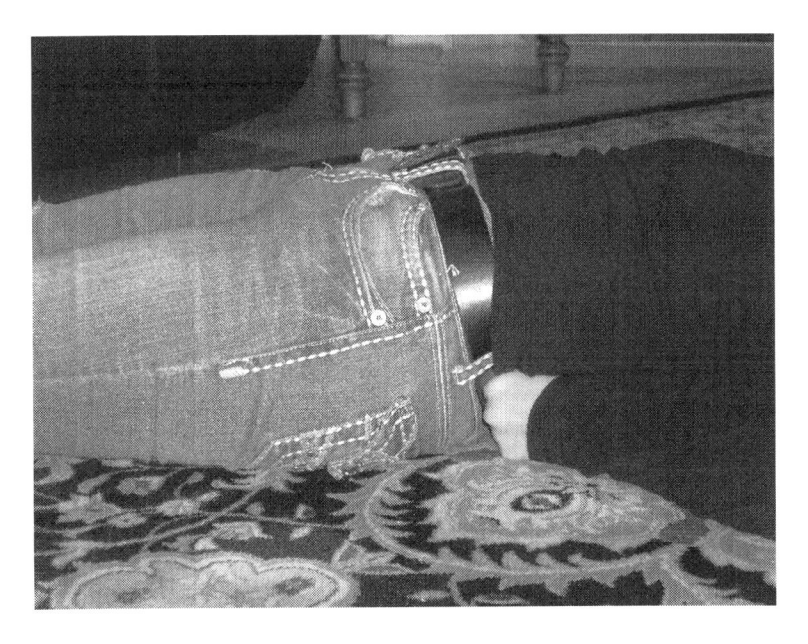

Blocking PSIS with Fist

Si Walking Adjustment

This is basically the same as the walking sacrum technique except for which bone you press on. The heel of the hand works best as shown in the photos because of the amount of pressure that is needed to affect the adjustment.

Some people can use the fingers, but this takes a fair amount of strength. A massage tool works better especially if you can't reach the bone.

This point can be hard to find, so feel around to be sure you have the PSIS. You can see the location in the photo above.

The action is to pull up from under the PSIS as you walk. Lengthen through the spine standing up tall as you walk taking five to eight steps.

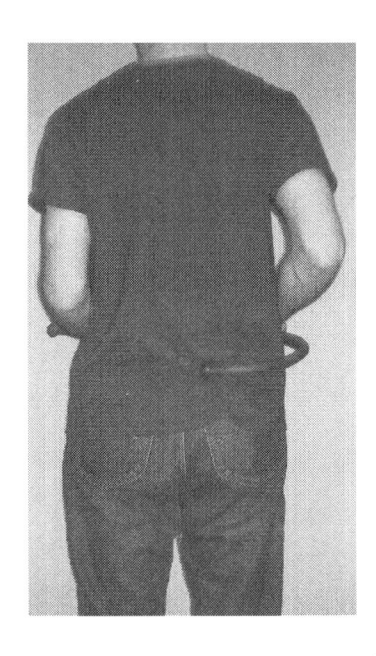

Hook the Massage Tool on the SI Joint

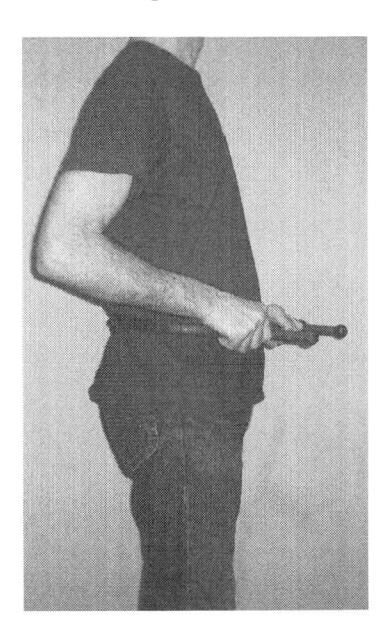

Pull the Massage Tool, Lengthen Through the Spine

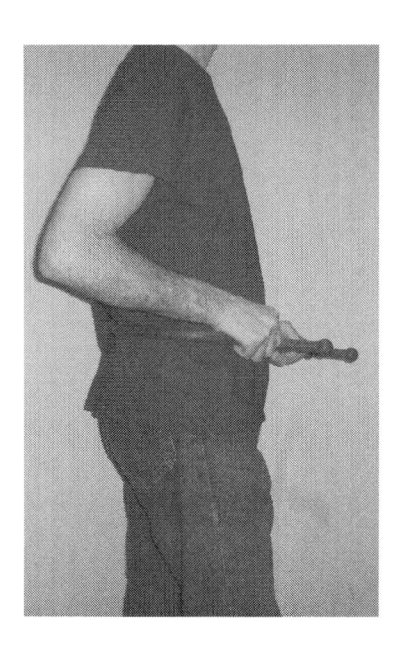

Keep Pressure on the SI Joint and Walk

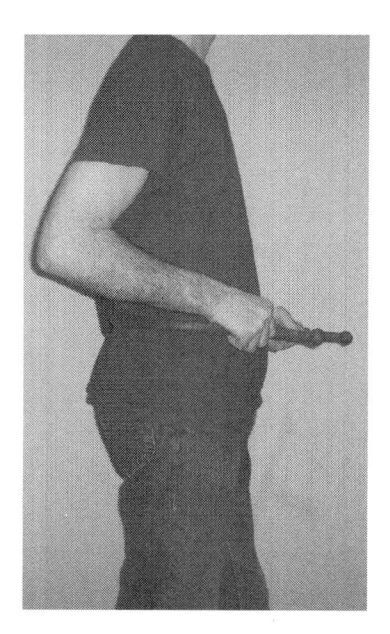

Keep Your Spine Tall as You Take Several Steps

Adjusting the Sit Bones

The sit bones or ischium are the bones you sit on. To find them, sit on a firm surface and reach under your bottom from the side and feel the bones that are supporting your weight.

When standing they are at the very bottom of the buttocks. They are about three inches apart for men, and three and a half to four inches apart for women. You can use your fingers to reach in and pull up on them while walking, or use the massage tool while walking. Lengthen through the spine as you take your five to eight steps.

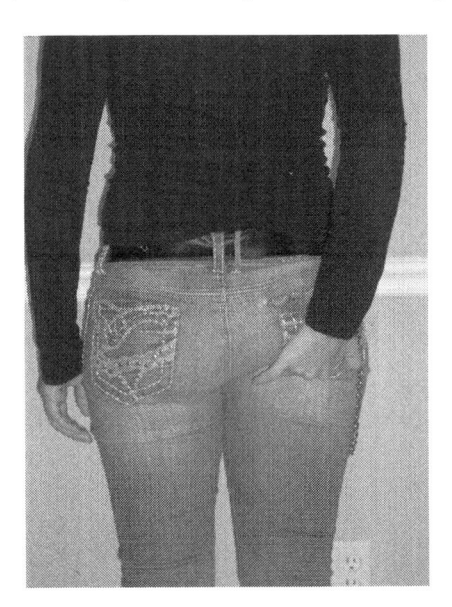

Find the Sit Bone at the Bottom of the Buttocks

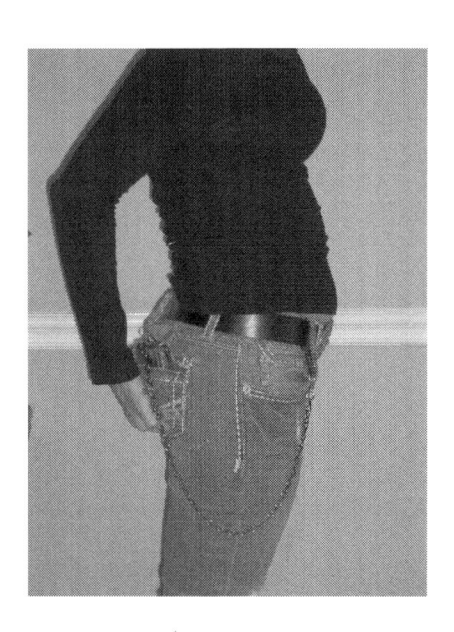

Pull Up on the Sit Bone to Rotate the Hip Structure Clockwise in this Photo

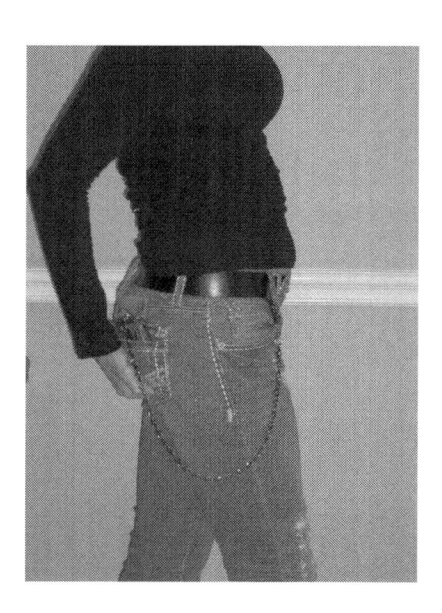

Walk While Pulling the Sit Bone Up, and Keeping the Spine Long

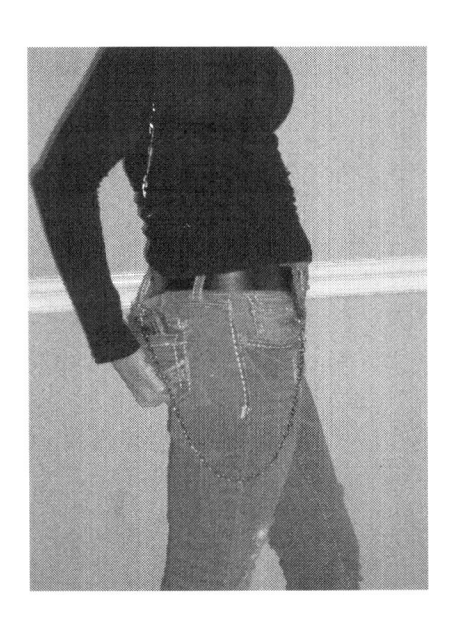

Continue Walking a Few Steps While Pulling Up

Using a massage tool to do the adjustment works better because it is easier to pull the sit bone up.

Notice that the male site bones are closer in than a woman's. This has to do with the difference in the width of the hips.

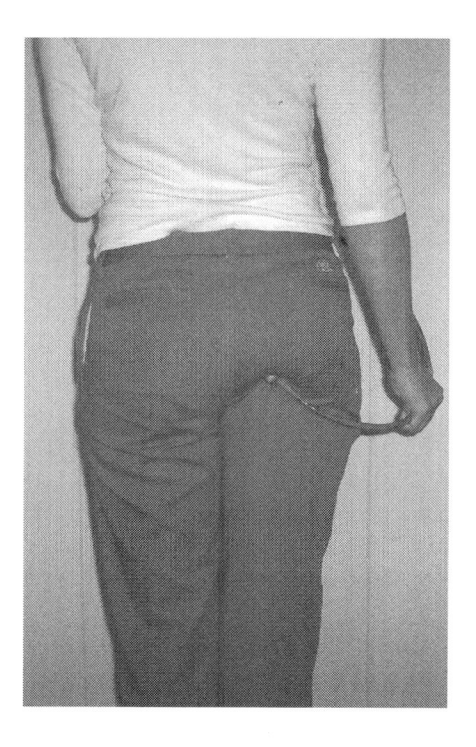

Pull Up On the Site Bone with a Massage Tool. Note the Closer in Position for the Man versus the Wider Spacing that a Woman's Hips Have.

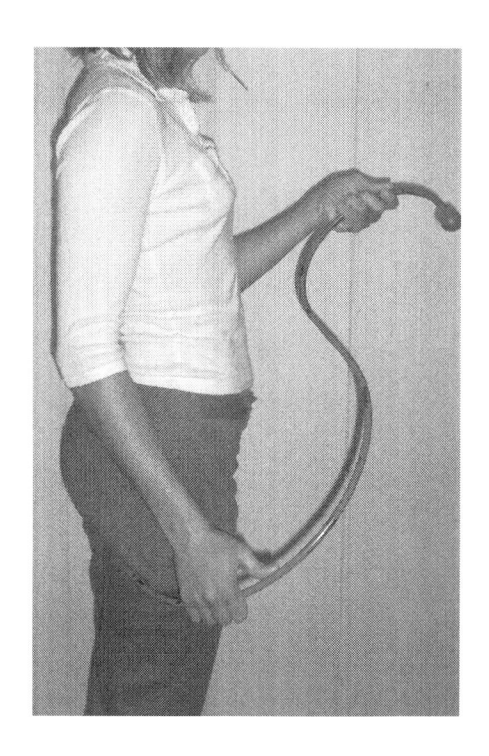

**Pull Up and Walk to Rotate the Hip Structure
Clockwise in this Photo**

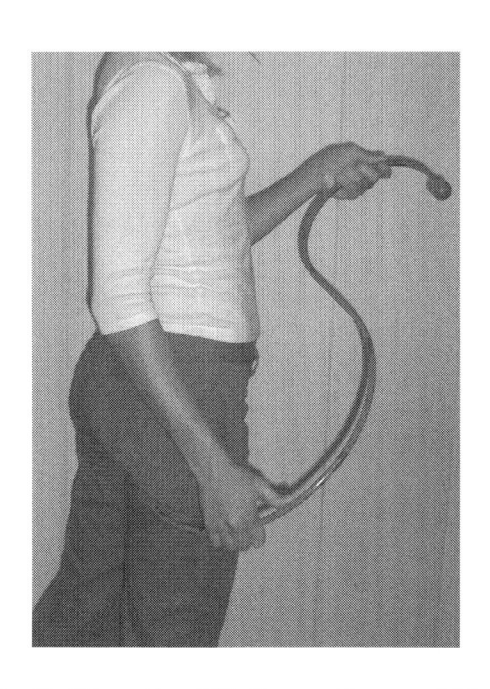

Walk While Pulling the Sit Bone Up, and Keeping the Spine Long

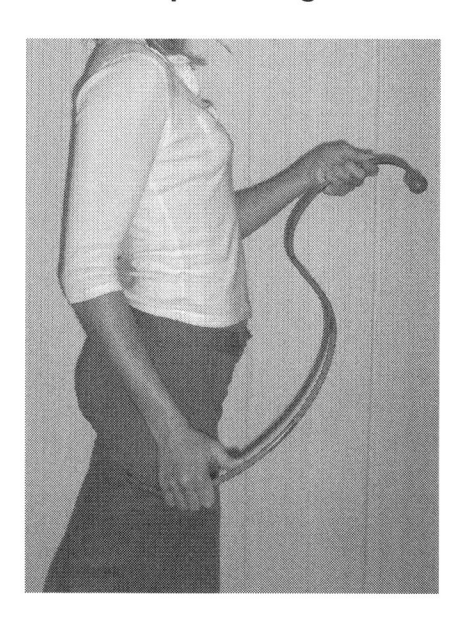

Continue Walking a Few Steps While Pulling Up

Sciatica

The sciatic nerve runs from the lower back down the back outer side of the thigh. Sciatica or pain in this nerve is usually a structural issue. It is also related to the piriformis muscle, a hip rotator at the top of the hip area. For some people the sciatic nerve runs through the piriformis while in most people it doesn't.

An inflamed piriformis is the primary cause of sciatica. But, a misalignment in the sacrum and the SI joint usually causes that inflammation. And, the bones themselves can cause direct pressure on the nerve causing the problem

Adjusting the sacrum, SI joint and ischium (sit bone) should relieve the pain, in many cases immediately. It can come back quickly though if the underlying issue is not corrected.

As with most structural issues, there may be a reason that the structure is out of alignment, so that may need to be addressed for long term relief. See the section on the adrenal glands to learn about the usual cause of the misalignment.

The Less Common SI Adjustment

If your lower back feels better when you arch your back and more uncomfortable when you round your back then you most likely need this adjustment.

This adjustment is done facing a wall or anything you can hold onto for balance. For the right side, take your right foot from behind with your right hand. Try to keep the right hip down and even with the left hip. It's okay if the hip comes up a little, but the higher the hip rises the less likely the adjustment will work. This will bring your back into an arch as you lift the leg which should feel good. If it doesn't feel good or at least ease the back pain, then stop, it is the wrong adjustment.

With a pumping action pull the foot and leg up and down several times. The back will likely loosen up and you will be able to pull the leg up higher and higher as you work it. Do this ten to twenty times, more if you like.

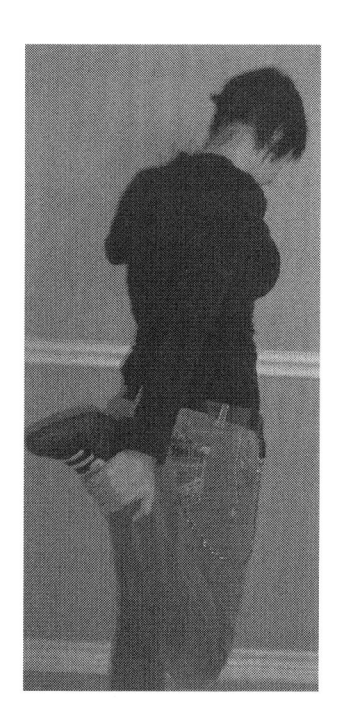

Draw the Back Leg Up while Holding a Wall

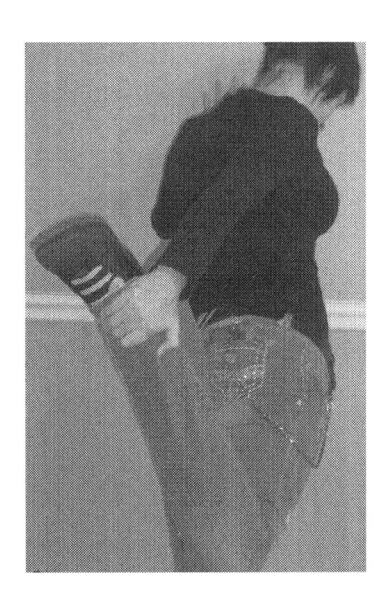

Pull the Back Leg Up and Down with a Pumping Action

Spinal Compression

The technical name for this is an imbrication. This happens when the vertebra in the lower back compress together. This can leave you feeling like things are jammed up in the lower back.

It is important to include this adjustment to completely adjust the lower back. Unfortunately, there is no effective way that I have found to do this adjustment yourself. However, it is possible to have someone do this adjustment on you. This is easy for someone who is strong and taller than you. It is possible for someone your height or slightly shorter than you to do the adjustment as long as they can pick you up.

Stand with your arms crossed, your right hand holding your left shoulder, and your left hand holding your right shoulder. Wrap your arms around tight enough so that your elbows are one on top of the other or close to it. Your friend stands behind you with their arms around you holding your elbows.

It works best if they squat down somewhat even if they are tall. You need to relax for this adjustment, so let your friend take most of your weight from the beginning. Take a deep breath and relax your body completely as you release the breath while your friend lifts you up off the floor and give you a downward shake with a little jerk at the end.

This pulls the spine long releasing the jam up in the vertebra. Sometimes many vertebras in the spine will pop at the same time, which usually feels pretty good.

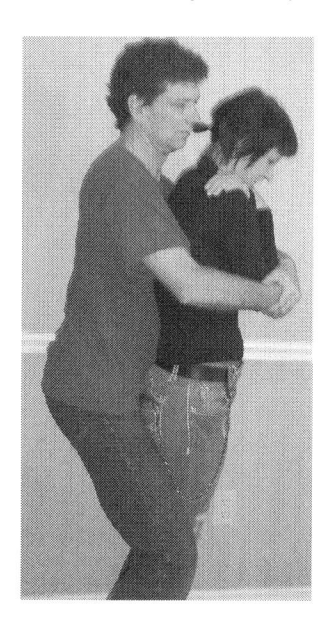

Cross Your Arms and Hold Your Shoulders. Your Helper Squats down Holding You by the Elbows

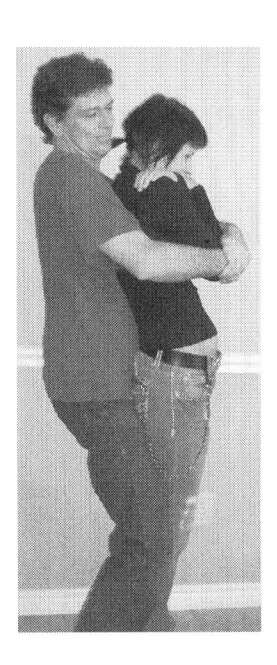

The Helper Picks You Up and Gives You a Shake Down

Muscle Testing

Most people will be able to easily find where to adjust and which way to adjust by feeling where the soreness is as described throughout the first part of this book. Muscle testing can also be used to find the specific area that is out and which way to adjust.

Muscle testing is becoming more and more popular these days as a technique to communicate with the body. Yes/no answers can be obtained on most any subject especially as it pertains to the body. Muscle testing is usually done with one person testing another. However, self-testing works for many people and substitute testing can be effective for someone that is injured, or not strong enough to be tested directly.

Muscle testing isn't as simple as the articles currently available make it seem. There are many things to know about muscle testing in order to get accurate results. Many of these accuracy techniques aren't known by most muscle testers. Muscle testing can be very frustrating with inaccurate results if these procedures aren't followed.

There are two main things you can do to insure an accurate test. The first is to drink a glass of water. Most people are dehydrated which makes testing difficult.

The other is to take a teaspoon of raw sesame seed oil. The reason is that there is a reversal having to do with birth trauma that causes inaccurate tests. The sesame seed oil fixes the problem and insures a more accurate test.

The following is from an article on my site, SelfAdjustingTechnique.com. There is more information available on the site. You can leave a comment there if you'd like to know more about the practice.

Muscle testing is a diagnostic tool that relies on the body's innate intelligence. When practiced by an accomplished muscle tester it is a good way to find out what is going on in the body. This article contains the basics of how to do a muscle test.

Muscle testing is not hard to do, however it does require some skill and practice. To practice, find a willing partner, perhaps someone that would also like to learn how to muscle test. For convenience, we will call the person being tested the client, and the one doing the test the practitioner.

Any muscle in the body can be used in muscle testing. The easiest muscle to learn on is the deltoid or shoulder muscle. Make sure your client's shoulder has some strength, and is uninjured. Avoid learning on someone that is really strong as very strong people can be difficult to test.

The Set Up
The easiest muscle to learn on is the deltoid or shoulder muscle. There are three muscles included in the deltoid. You have to isolate the one muscle in the group that you are going to test. If the client holds their arm straight out to the side you would be testing the lateral or side deltoid. If they hold their arm straight out in front you would be testing the anterior or front deltoid. Either of these are good for learning.

The best position to learn how to muscle test is standing. Alternately, your client can lie on their back with the test arm held up overhead.

Since you only want to use one muscle to test, have your

client hold their arm straight out to the side or directly out in front. If the arm is somewhere between the two positions you will be testing both the anterior and lateral deltoid. It is very difficult to test when more than one muscle is engaged.

Also, the arm must be held straight; if there is a bend at the elbow other muscles are being recruited which makes testing difficult or impossible. If the shoulder gets tired or sore they can switch to the other arm or with the arm held out in front.

It is best to learn using your dominant arm. For this we will consider that the practitioner is right handed. Adjust if you are left handed.

The Basic Method
Have your client stand facing you with their left arm held horizontally and straight out to their left side. Stand in front of them with your right hand palm down on their left arm just above the wrist. Put your left hand on the client's right shoulder to stabilize them. Keep your right hand open, if you grasp the arm you will affect the test.

Instruct your client to resist when you push on their arm. They should resist, but not fight against you as you push down on their arm. Start with a small amount of pressure and gradually increase until the arm starts to bend down. Since different people will be able to resist different amounts of pressure, this will show you how much you need to push to test this client

Release the pressure and test again, this time before you test say aloud, "show me a no." The arm should go all the way down when you apply roughly the same or even less pressure than you did before. Be sure to follow through keeping the pressure steady on their arm as you push down.

Repeat this time saying, 'show me a yes.' The arm should stay strong this time.

Keep practicing this yes/no test until you get clear results each time. Then try the test while thinking the instruction.

Caution
Be careful not to jerk down on your client's test arm. This is a common mistake and will not produce accurate results. It could even result in an injury to your client.

Conclusion
This is the basic method for doing a muscle test. It takes practice to do good muscle testing so keep practicing. Try not to be too discouraged by poor results, it takes practice.

Muscle Testing a Joint

To test a particular joint all you need to do is touch or have your client touch the joint and test the muscle. If their muscle goes weak then there is something up with the joint. You can confirm by testing again with the statement "this joint is out of alignment."

Next you can test which direction it is out by making the statement "this joint is rotated to the right side." Any variation that is similar to this will work.

The main thing is to make statements. Questions do not work very well in muscle testing. Testing a statement as true or not, a strong or weak muscle is the only method that works correctly.

The Adrenal Glands

Earlier I mentioned energy systems in the body that affect the well-being of the lower back. One of the main energy systems are the adrenal glands. These are two walnut sized glands that sit on top of the kidneys. That's what adrenal means, adjacent to the renal which means kidney.

In traditional Chinese medicine, low kidney chi is roughly related to the strength and functionality of the adrenal glands though they don't really look at it the way most naturopathic practitioners do. Adrenal fatigue is a very common condition affecting almost every client I see.

These little glands produce a quart (liter) of hormones every day! They use a lot of vitamin B6, pantothenic acid, vitamin C, B12 and niacin amide to do this. These are the same nutrients that the ligaments and tendons need to stay healthy and strong.

Adrenal hormones are more important to homeostasis or chemical balance in the body than ligaments and tendons. When the adrenal glands are overworked the needed nutrients are preferentially supplied to them leaving the ligaments and tendons weak from the lack of nutrition. The lower back is usually the first area to be affected by this lack of nutrition because of the amount of weight they support.

I like to think of it as the body saying, "slow down and take it easy, you're pushing too hard." This is almost impossible for most people in this busy modern world. The stress of fulfilling our obligations prevents us from taking time off just because our back hurts.

One of the stress factors are emotional in nature, which

results in low adrenal strength which can cause lower back pain.

In the US, many back surgeries are done for lower back pain with a very low rate of full recovery. In Europe lower back pain is more often treated with rest with a much higher rate of full recovery.

The above information gives us an obvious treatment for lower back pain; take some time off and allow the adrenal glands to recover and the back will get better, at least more often than with drugs and aggressive treatment.

Another common cause of adrenal fatigue is caffeine. Caffeine depletes the adrenal glands directly. Whether it's coffee, tea, green tea or, heaven forbid, caffeinated sodas.

Caffeine causes the adrenal glands to release large amounts of hormones like cortisol and adrenaline. The pickup you feel from caffeine is adrenaline making your heart beat faster.

Some people's adrenal glands have been so drained by overuse that they don't get a rise from caffeine anymore. The adrenal glands just don't have anything left to put out.

The main reason for adrenal fatigue and therefore lower back pain is the modern diet. The modern diet is completely opposite to how our ancient ancestors ate.

Recently, relatively new technology has shown that 200,000 years ago and beyond the diet of our ancestors consisted of ninety percent animal protein. If you look in the supermarket, about ninety percent of the contents are highly processed foods.
That is what the modern diet is for most people, ninety

percent processed foods. The complete opposite of what our ancestors ate, the way our bodies developed over eons.

I'm not endorsing a diet of mostly animal protein. A balanced diet of vegetables, fruits, animal protein and whole grains is what works best.

Sugar and processed foods are the main cause of most modern ailments like heart disease, cancer, depression, Alzheimer's disease, chronic fatigue, diabetes and more.

Processed foods put incredible stress on the adrenal glands causing them to become depleted. Following is an explanation of the pathway for processed foods and sugar affecting adrenal health and how that affects the lower back.

This is only the beginning of the story though. There are several different pathways that result in these much more serious conditions. But, that is for another time.

Sugar of any kind, caffeine and alcohol are absorbed directly into the blood from the stomach. Alcohol is just highly concentrated sugar. When sugar absorbs quickly into the blood the blood sugar levels go up very quickly.

Whole grains and vegetables are complex carbohydrates which break down slowly. Their sugars are released slowly in the small intestines which results in a slow rise in blood sugar.

Any ground up grain is a processed food. These processed grains are ground down into a fine powder which leaves more surface area exposed so that they digest faster. Processed grains and sugar are called simple carbohydrates because they digest faster and release sugar much faster than whole grains.

Whole grains means not cut up as in steel cut oats, or ground up into flour. All ground up grains digest quickly, whether the brain layer is left or not. That means that foods like whole wheat bread release sugar into the blood almost as fast as white bread or white rice. The main point is that sugar and refined grains bring blood sugar levels up too high and too fast.

High blood sugar levels cause the body to release high levels of insulin. Insulin is the mechanism in the body that brings blood sugar down. Continuous high levels of insulin eventually degrade or break down the insulin receptor sites on the cell walls. This is insulin resistance or type 2 diabetes, or chronic high blood sugar.

The less effective insulin is the more insulin is produced by the pancreas. The pancreas can burn out if this continues long enough. A non-functioning pancreas means that there is no insulin at all to bring down the blood sugar resulting in a need for regular insulin injections or type 1 diabetes.

High levels of insulin cause many biochemical reactions in the body, more than the scope of this book. Suffice to say that a high level of insulin is the start of most major ailments today. This includes many types of cancer, heart disease, diabetes, depression and many other conditions that were very rare before World War Two and the advent of processed foods.

People often argue that we enjoy a longer life span in this modern world with modern medicine. This is true, but the main reason for that is sanitation. Until only recently the leading causes of human death were pathogenic infections.

The water wasn't safe to drink, and simple infections very often led to death. Today we take antibiotics and take clean water for granted. If we get sick we just go to the doctor for a prescription and everything is better.

Accidents and injuries were the secondary causes of death. Modern medicine is excellent at repairing an injured body. Childbirth was a major risk to both mother and child.

Today, even though we do live longer, the quality of those later years is highly questionable with all the modern diseases that plague us.

Another little bit of biochemistry for you to contemplate; all this sugar has to go somewhere. One place it goes is into fat cells for storage via the liver where it is first converted into triglycerides, the form it needs to be in for fat storage. Consequently, the main causes of cholesterol issues are excess blood sugar and high levels of insulin.

So, why is high blood sugar so bad for the back? Suppose you eat a candy bar or a pastry. Your energy will shoot up really high for a half hour or so. This is the high blood sugar we've been talking about. After that, you crash and get sleepy which happens because of the body's insulin over reaction which drives the blood sugar down too low.

If you don't re-dose with sugar, the low blood sugar will cause you to be lethargic for an hour or so, maybe you would even take a nap. It will probably be hard to do much of anything during that recovery time. Even thinking can be difficult. This is because the brain uses mostly sugar. When the blood sugar is low the brain is starved causing this lethargy.

Later, you will start to feel a little more normal again. This is because the low blood sugar causes the adrenal glands to release cortisol which brings the blood sugar back up to normal. You feel normal again.

One of the problems with this kind of sugar consumption is that people often re-dose with sugar to keep the energy levels up so that they feel good. Of course, this causes the blood sugar to bounce up and down as long as the sugar consumption continues. This results in the release of more and more insulin and cortisol.

This constant demand on the adrenal glands causes them to become weakened. Overworked, they swell in their attempt to keep up with this constant demand. The constant onslaught of processed foods like bread, pasta, corn chips, fruit juice, dried fruit and sugar keep them working harder than their capacity.

Eventually they become drained causing many intense symptoms including lower back pain because of the adrenal glands demand for the same nutrients as ligaments and tendons. Other symptoms of adrenal fatigue are listed below.

Each of the above compensations are the body's normal response to stress. The body is designed to deal with stress in this way from thousands of years of dealing with the demands of survival in the ancient world, including the stress of sugar consumption.

For example, we crave sugar because our ancient ancestors had to fatten up on the ripe fruits at the end of summer to create a reserve so they could survive the lack of food in the winter. The insulin response was necessary for fattening up at the end of the growing season. Type 2 diabetes is a natural reaction that we had to have in order to fatten up, but only once a year.

Our modern problem is that treats are available all the time, so we are always fattening up! Type 2 diabetes becomes chronic.

To summarize, high intake of sugar in the form of processed foods and sugar causes excess insulin to release into the blood. Insulin levels that are too high bring blood sugar levels down too low. The compensation for this is the release of cortisol by the adrenal glands to bring the blood sugar back up again. This constant bouncing around of the blood sugar eventually exhausts the adrenal glands in their attempt to keep blood sugar levels normal.

Similar problems happen when you go hungry. Blood sugar drops from the lack of calories. So, the adrenal glands release cortisol to keep the blood sugar up. Cortisol is a stress hormone and not eating is stressful for the body. This is why starvation diets where meals are skipped rarely work.

Of course, it's a little more complex than that. The hypothalamus, the pituitary and the adrenal glands form a circuit called the HPA axis which will bring the pancreas where insulin is produced into the mix. These glands work together to keep blood sugar balanced.

Communication between these glands is mostly via hormone secretions with much of this information going to the brain via Vagus nerve causing the problem at C5 that was discussed earlier in the section on C5.

Further analysis of how this involves other systems in the body reveals how major illnesses result from excess blood sugar, the resulting excess insulin and the body working to compensate.

As you can see from all of this, the best thing you can do for your adrenal glands is to stop eating processed foods like sugar and ground up grains. Pretty much anything that comes in a package will have one or both of these ingredients. Many restaurants use a lot of processed foods, so you have to be mindful there as well.

Symptoms of Adrenal Fatigue

Adrenal fatigue is one of the most common conditions that people suffer from today. Mostly it is because of the modern diet and the ready availability of processed foods. All these great snacks that are always available are just too hard to resist!

Unfortunately, our bodies are designed to desire sweet foods as a necessary survival trait. Even the strongest willed have trouble resisting sweets and other processed foods.

There are many symptoms of adrenal fatigue. Just because you have one or more of these symptoms doesn't necessarily mean that you have adrenal fatigue though. Some of these symptoms can be caused by other factors.

Contra-wise, just because you don't have any of these symptoms, or the symptom is minor doesn't mean that you don't have adrenal fatigue. In most cases of adrenal fatigue there will probably be several of these symptoms, or you could have just one.

50 Symptoms of Adrenal Fatigue

1. Excessive fatigue and exhaustion, chronic fatigue
2. Non-refreshing sleep
3. Sleep disturbance, insomnia
4. Feeling overwhelmed or unable to cope
5. Craving salty

6. Sensitivity to light
7. Low stamina and slow to recover from exercise
8. Slow to recover from injury or illness
9. Difficulty concentrating
10. Poor digestion
11. Irritable bowel syndrome, IBS
12. Low immune function
13. Premenstrual syndrome
14. Menopause symptoms
15. Low blood pressure
16. Sensitivity to cold
17. Fearfulness
18. Allergies
19. Frequent influenza
20. Arthritis
21. Anxiety
22. Irritability
23. Depression
24. Poor memory
25. Low libido, sexual drive or interest
26. Lack of lust for life and/or food
27. Excess hunger
28. Low appetite
29. Panic/anxiety attacks
30. Irritability, impatience, quick to anger
31. Lower back pain
32. Brain fog
33. Dramatic mood shift
34. Infertility
35. Chronic stress and related health issues
36. Chronically being "on edge"
37. Skin problems
38. Diarrhea
39. Muscle and joint pain
40. Hypoglycemia
41. Waking in the night, trouble getting back to sleep.
42. Migraine headaches
43. Osteoporosis

44. Low body temperature, thyroid issue
45. Rapid aging
46. Afternoon tiredness
47. Thinning hair or hair loss
48. Caffeine fails to energize
49. Craving sweets and junk food
50. Frequent infections

Adrenal Fatigue Tests

There are several tests that can be done to determine if your adrenal glands are fatigued. There are laboratories that examine saliva samples to accurately tell you the levels of hormones in the blood which will reveal the state of the adrenal glands. While these tests are worthwhile, they are expensive and take time. However, there are simple tests that don't cost anything at all. And, you get immediate results.

A really easy self-test can be done with a mirror and a flashlight. Have the room dim, but light enough that you can see your pupils in the mirror. Notice how the pupils are dilated or large.

Shine the flashlight into one eye from the side so that you can still see your pupil in the mirror, but so that the light is still bright enough to cause the pupil to shrink down. If your adrenal glands are healthy, your pupils will immediately shrink to a pinpoint. If your adrenal glands are weak, there will be a lag before they reduce in size.

Keep shining the light and watching your pupil for at least a minute or two to see if they hold the contraction.

Now you know why adrenal fatigue often causes sensitivity to light.

The postural blood pressure test tests the way adrenal glands respond to the less blood going to the upper body when you stand up. Healthy adrenal glands put out a little adrenaline when you stand up so the pressure stays steady preventing the lightheadedness that sometimes happens from standing quickly.

The first thing you do is to lie down for ten minutes or so and relax. Then take your BP noting the numbers. For this test, you want to pay attention to the lower number called the diastolic.

Next, stand up and take the BP again right away. If the diastolic drops by five or ten points then your adrenals are fatigued.

Take the pressure again after three minutes or so to see if the pressure recovers to the level it was while reclining. If not, then the stress the adrenals have been living with is still present and they are not recovering.

The only things that will help are lifestyle changes, herbs and supplements. If it stays at the same lower reading after a few minute of standing then the adrenal glands are still weak, but recovering.

A last test is to palpate, or feel the adrenal glands directly. The adrenal glands become inflamed when they are stressed because they are trying harder and harder to keep up with demand.

You are actually going to be feeling the lymphatics that are related to the adrenal glands. They are located one inch up and one inch out from the bellybutton. Press in a couple of inches or more and feel around as their location will vary slightly from person to person. Feel for them one at a time.

One will usually be more inflamed than the other if there is a problem. They are not very hard to find if they are inflamed though you may have to press in somewhat especially if there is fatty tissue in the way. They can be somewhat difficult to find, so take your time and be thorough.

If they are fatigued, they will feel swollen and there is usually a very uncomfortable feeling or it can hurt. Healthy adrenal lymphatics can be found, but you will have to press in even deeper. If they are healthy they won't mind the pressure too much, that is it won't hurt or be very uncomfortable at all.

Treatment for the Adrenal Glands

As stated above, the ligaments and tendons are in competition with the adrenal glands for nutrition with the adrenal glands taking the lions share. This results in a depletion that can result in much of the lower back pain that people often experience.

The nutrients that will help are B6, pantothenic acid, vitamin C, niacin amide, and B12. There are other factors that the adrenal glands use, but these are the main ones. Taking these nutrients will help the adrenal glands.

One thing that needs to be understood about vitamins in general is that they are useless in the body unless they are first activated by enzymes. The body produces most of these enzymes, but there is an issue with B6 where the body doesn't produce its coenzyme. Consequently, there is a worldwide epidemic of B6 deficiency due this enzyme deficiency. I won't go into the reason for this now, but I bet that if you start taking the enzyme activated form of B6 that you will notice a difference in how you feel.

The chemical name for enzyme activated B6 is pyridoxal 5 phosphate or P5P. This has become available in many health food stores in the US. They usually come in 50 mg tablets though sometimes the label says something lower, around 35 mg. This can be confusing, but they are generally the same. I recommend that you start with two or three twice a day.

When you get niacin amide, be sure you aren't getting niacin. Niacin causes a flush that can be pretty uncomfortable, and really isn't very good for you either. I recommend 500 mg each of niacin amide and pantothenic acid in the morning with food, and 6 grams (6000 mg) calcium ascorbate per day spread out throughout the day.

I like calcium ascorbate because it won't cause diarrhea like ascorbic acid can, and it isn't hard on the kidneys like ascorbic acid.

B12 is good for general energy issues. The dosage will vary, but a good dose to start with is 500 mcg per day.

There are other products that are better for treating the adrenal glands, but they are more costly. My favorite protocol is a combination of herbs and supplements that are available through Standard Process.

Herbs and supplements that are available through Standard Process are not generally available to the public. They want people to have a trained practitioner dispense the products because the wrong ones can cause harm. Consequently, you may have to find a practitioner to buy them though many are available online.

MediHerb is a very high quality product that is far superior to just about any tincture or herb that you will find in the health food stores. The only other herbs that I know of that are as good are Kroeger Herbs.

Here is the primary protocol for weakened adrenal glands.

Drenatrophin PMG - 3 twice a day
Cataplex B - 3 twice a day
Cataplex C - 4 twice a day
Eleuthero Liquid - 11 ml per day
Licorice High Grade Liquid - 4 ml per day

The herbs should be taken morning and around noon as they can affect sleep. On an empty stomach is best, but take them with food if you have trouble remembering.

Alternate protocol for high blood pressure

Drenamine - 4 twice a day
Cataplex B - 2 in the morning and 1 in the evening
Eleuthero Liquid - 11 ml per day
Rehmannia - 5 ml per day

The above are protocols are not advised for pregnant or nursing women. It is better to use this one:

Pantothenic Acid: 500 mg in the morning
Niacin Amide: 500 mg in the morning
Vitamin C: 1000 mg twice a day
Bioflavonoids: 500 mg twice a day
B12 as Cyanocobalamin: at least 1000 mcg in the morning

Enzyme activated B6 (pyridoxal-5-phosphate): 100 mg in the morning and 50 mg in the evening. Need may actually be more, up to 250 mg per day in two or three doses. See note on B6 below.

Alternate Adrenal Protocol

This is a good protocol as well. It is sometimes better depending on the individual. It has the added benefit of being mostly topical creams for people who have a problem taking pills.

They are from Apex Energetics. Follow the instructions on the containers. If you don't experience the results you expect then you might consider increasing the dosage.

The topical creams are Adrena Calm, and Adrena Stim. Apply them to an area of the skin that has no hair for the best absorption. Adapto Crine is a capsule. Take it on an empty stomach if you can remember, with food if you need that reminder.

I would also recommend taking fish oils or some other form of omega three fatty acids from animal sources. They are the bodies only natural anti-inflammatory and can help reduce the inflammation that usually comes with back pain.

Plant source omega-3 fatty acids don't have the same effect because they have to go through a lot of steps to be used as anti-inflammatories. As a result they usually get used for something else along the way.

You will be deficient in omega-3 fatty acids if you don't eat fish regularly. You can start with a fairly high dose of three to six 1000 mg capsules twice a day for a month or so. Reduce it to one or two capsules twice a day within two months though because a long term high dosage can be hard on the gallbladder.

There are other herbs and supplements that work really well too. There is so much variability with these though that it is best to use these with consultation.

Traditional Chinese medicine is another good modality for treating the adrenal glands. I have found that people respond much better to acupuncture and herbs if they also eliminate grains for a few weeks. And of course, eliminate sugar, alcohol and caffeine.

Another factor that can help the adrenal glands heal is detoxification. There are many detoxification techniques and programs available. For now, find one that suits you and stick to it. You can look on my website to find more information about detoxification.

If you want to know more about adrenal fatigue and what you can do about it for yourself you can get my book Adrenal Fatigue -- Get Your Life Back. It has a lot more information on the subject that you will likely find useful.

Conclusion

Most people can successfully use Self Adjusting Technique to adjust their own back, neck, hips and ribs. The pain and complications of traditional chiropractic adjustments can be avoided with simple and gentle self-treatment. Some method of dealing with stress and emotional issues that are at the root of the misalignment may be needed. Chronic lower back pain and sciatica will usually require time, lifestyle changes, herbs and supplements.

The good news is that now there are ways to treat these conditions with minimal cost. Most if not all of this can be done with the information found in this book. I wish you every success in the use of these techniques.

Contact Me

If you ever need help working out how to do an adjustment you can contact me through my website. You might also like to sign up for my newsletter. You don't have to worry about spam either as I will never sell or rent your email address.

There are methods of strengthening the ligaments and tendons and muscles associated with different joints so that they will hold an adjustment better. And, there are methods of dealing with much of the stress and emotional issues that we all have. Visit my website where you will find a contact form.

About Kalidasa

Kalidasa is a yoga teacher and natural healer based in the San Francisco Bay Area. He has been a successful yoga teacher since 1980 working with thousands of people over the years. His ability is widely acknowledged among his many students and yoga teachers alike.

He used his knowledge of the body to develop Self Adjusting Technique. This process started in 1993 and still continues as he finds more and easier methods to facilitate gentle adjustments.

In 1995 he started studying natural healing, biochemistry, nutrition and Applied Kinesiology from a master healer. Shortly after he began his studies he began treating friends with surprising success.

He considered this practice, but his results were such that his natural healing practice grew quickly. His healing ability is highly acclaimed by his clients and piers which include medical doctors, acupuncturists, homeopaths, nutritionists, chiropractors and others.

You can find more information on his website at http://SelfAdjustingTechnique.com. His site has many articles on natural healing, information that you can use to help heal yourself of various conditions. His goal is to make natural healing available to everyone at minimal cost.

Made in the USA
Lexington, KY
03 December 2012